STAYING BALANCED

AFTER WEIGHT LOSS

SURGERY

15 TIPS FOR SUCCESS

A.E. McKay

If you or anyone you know has ever tried to lose weight and keep it off, you already understand the drill: diet, exercise and wait - yes, wait...until you have to do it over and over again. Many people feel that diet and exercise is just a part of life, but to a food addict, this is more like a horror show. Enduring weight loss is chock full of trials and tribulations fraught with pain and suffering and most often it leaves the food addict psychologically, physically and spiritually damaged when the weight comes back on - usually within a couple of months after a diet. I'm not here to communicate with people who are 15, 20, 25 or even 40 pounds overweight. I'm speaking now to people that, for years, have struggled with the emotional aspects of being a food addict and are at least 50 to 75 pounds or more overweight. Is this you? If so, I hope you will carefully read these tips from someone who has been there and understands what you are going through in your struggles.   This book is for people who suffer from an emotional addiction to food. For folks like me that have already admitted this, we have been able to use our pain to regain our power and to stay balanced and life a new, healthy lifestyle.

This may be difficult for you to admit right now but it's imperative that before we can talk openly about the *success* and the various ways to achieve this, anyone reading must be willing and open to the possibilities that they have an addiction to food *that is emotional and this has created obstacles in their lives for which they have protected themselves with very visible layers* - the excess weight that shows on the outside is what is carefully guarding our hearts and minds from past and present pain.

I already know, you've tried everything. You've listed to family, friends, medical professionals and countless others telling you that you must lose weight. These helpful people have informed you your health is suffering and if you don't do something soon, you will die or your quality of life will suffer.

I can't tell you how many people told me this when I was at the height of despair in my life. People told me this, I think, hoping they could help. Clearly, when I couldn't walk up a flight of stairs without being winded and had to sleep with a C-Pap at night as I stopped breathing so many times due to Sleep Apnea, I already knew I was in crisis. Your family and friends are trying to be loving and helpful.

Believe me, their hearts are in the right place and they *do* mean well. Unfortunately, many think that the *tough love* approach is the best way to attack the situation but a food addict's mind is different. The bitter irony is that food is the manifestation of our inner pain and suffering and is what we are carrying around with us for the world to see.

The real truth is that until YOU are ready to change, there is not anything that will happen to make your life different. It's all in your mind and if your mind isn't buying this life-altering change, nothing (not even something as radical as medical weight loss surgery) will work. Always keep this in mind because it has never left my conscious thought since March of 2008 when I had surgery.

When I had weight loss surgery, I had tried every possible diet imaginable for over 20 years, been on weight loss medication supervised by my doctor, attended classes on obesity, gone to Weight Watchers multiple times and Jenny Craig. I tried NutriSystem, Richard Simmons (both his Sweatin' to the Oldies and his Food Mover Program), read about 25 books on every diet from The South Beach Diet to Atkins and never had any long term success.

Why? Because I was treating only one symptom (really the byproduct) of my food addiction: my weight gain. That's what most of us do to survive in a society that conditions us to be thin. The diet, fitness and wellness industry is a multi-billion industry (tied in with fashion and beauty) that tells us we are never good enough. These industries tell us to be healthy, keep fit and then you can wear beautiful clothes that look stunning.

From a very early age, everything that surrounds us in media and advertisements tells us to be thin and wear nice clothes for people to look at us! I'm certain there are many people who may read this and they will laugh. *I guarantee all food addicts secretly have that one outfit that we would love to wear someday* when we are thin. We buy it knowing it won't fit but secretly hoping for the day it does. And it sits in our closet year after year until we eventually buy another one to take its place. I did this all the time until I couldn't shop anymore at regular stores and needed to shop online or at shops for bigger people. *Clothes will not fix your problems. Your issues are emotional and will remain until you make a commitment to change your life.*

Deciding to have Medical Weight Loss Surgery is a major life decision. If you are thinking about surgery, it means you, like millions of others throughout the world, are at your wit's end trying to cope with being heavy. For some it is vanity (i.e. I want to be thin so others will notice me), for others it's necessity (i.e. if I don't lose weight I will die) and for others it is a combination of wanting to make a life change and shed all of the excess weight as a plan to be able to do something they haven't been able to do because of the weight (i.e. care for a child or loved one, take a trip, etc.).

I remember I wanted to go Ziplining, you know, where you hang on a wire and go from point to point in a forest. At 330, I was well over the 250 pound maximum weight limit. I also never again wanted to shop at Big and Tall or wear a seat belt extender on an airplane. Perhaps those reasons seem vain to some but the shame for me was unbearable as I travelled for work and just hated the look on passenger's faces when the heavy me walked down the aisle and got a middle seat on a late Friday afternoon flight.

Just because you are considering surgery doesn't mean you need to have it. I chose this option carefully and mostly because I knew I was at a life stage where I was in my 40's and if I didn't do this now my quality of life by my 50's would be non-existent or I would be dead. Your journey is *yours*, please know that others do care but in the end the choice to have a surgical procedure is yours. Just as is the type of procedure you will have or consider. Don't let doctors, friends, loved ones or anyone push you into weight loss surgery- this is a life-altering event and if you are not properly educated on the consequences, it can lead to disaster.

You will hear from everyone against weight loss surgery who say the same thing: just diet and exercise. I wish I had a dollar for everyone that said this to me as I would be rich. *It's an addiction.* You cannot just diet and exercise just like the drug addict or alcoholic can't just use or drink a *little.* Insidious as it is, *our* addiction to food is horrible since we must eat to exist. Without food we would die. Yet, eating too much food, we will *also* die. It's in learning to balance our lives where we can regain control and start a new life.

These 15 Tips can be used for the food addict who is considering surgery, someone who is trying to reclaim their body, has had surgery and for those that are currently struggling with weight issues.

These tips are about life and life balance most of all. The weight WILL come off, but if you are not balanced or prepared, there will be consequences (often tragic ones) which I can personally attest to and *do* happen.

By now, you probably have already done some very extensive and careful research on the Weight Loss Clinic, Hospital and Surgical Team you will select. Hopefully, you have been approved for coverage for this type of procedure by your insurance company and medically cleared to have the procedure.

These three things are vital and until you have a surgeon you trust, have the approval for payment by your insurance and you are healthy enough to have a medical procedure, nothing else matters.

If you are looking for a surgeon or weight loss clinic, you will want to search for Bariatric Surgery (the clinical term).

Most reputable surgeons and hospitals hold monthly informational seminars to learn about all the different procedures for weight loss surgery as there are several. They have other former patients that attend who have gone through the procedures and these people are available to talk to you afterwards.

It's extremely important you like the team you will be working with and know all the upfront costs as well as costs you will incur down the road. *Weight Loss surgery is not cheap.* Most addictions are not cheap if you really think about it.

You will incur many costs along the way, not the least of these being several new wardrobes (think a new set of clothes for every 40 or 50 pounds as a rule of thumb) and you will understand what I mean.

For example, I was a XXL with a 52 inch waist that went to a Medium and a 32 inch waist over 3 years and have settled on Large and 34 inch waist now at 6 years so you might imagine the wardrobe it takes for personal *and* work attire.

Even your shoe size can change in the most bizarre way as the soles of your feed have fat so shoes don't always fit the same after losing a large amount of weight.

As far as Insurance Payment for the various procedures go, it's a total crapshoot. Every plan is different and it is total insanity what different plans will pay for and what other plans will not.

I had a nightmare the first time I tried to have surgery in 2006 as I was told insurance would pay but I had to get it approved after 6 months of a medically supervised weight loss program and all these other courses and tests I had to have (psychological assessment, 3 classes on weight loss) and oh, yeah, I had to lose 10% of my excess body weight before surgery! After I did all this, I could then apply to get it approved by insurance. Looking back, jumping through all these hoops seemed cruel as I needed help just like someone needing rehab. I needed food addict rehab!

Guess what? Yep, they denied the procedure! After six months on Phentermine for weight loss, losing 30 pounds, taking all the classes I was denied the surgery. I appealed the decision but ended up moving out of state to start a new life.

Four months later (and after I left my job and didn't purchase COBRA insurance benefits since my new company paid for insurance) I got a letter that my appeal was *approved* for the surgery.

Unfortunately, my new insurance didn't cover the procedure at all so over the next two years between 2006-2008 I gained back the 30 pounds and added another 30 pounds more just for the heck of it. Have you ever done something like this yourself that was self-destructive?

Almost a year and a half later, a TV commercial came on talking about the St. Francis Hospital Medical Weight Loss Program in Federal Way, Washington (about thirty minutes South of Seattle). It was a Center of Excellence which in the medical field is a program that has gone through extensive processes for approval for a procedure. They specialized in the Lap Band and traditional Roux-en-Y Gastric Bypass surgeries but also performed others not as common.

I had switched insurance companies again but they still didn't cover the procedure. They only would cover the pre-operative testing (go figure).

The surgery cost over $20,000 plus the medical tests which were about $5,000. Thanks to my Mom and savings, I decided to forget insurance and pay for it all myself.

I'm spending time describing this as it is extremely important you take a reality check here - this is *expensive*. It is worth it? *Yes.* Would I do it again? Absolutely, without question. It cost me literally most of my savings.

My dear mother told me she loved me and wanted me to live which gave me such a boost. If that isn't a reason to keep the weight off after surgery, I don't know what other testimonial there is in life.

I strongly encourage that if you have funds and can pay that you should pay rather than waiting. Things have improved over the past ten years but all the hoops you need to go through are discouraging at best. It's your call, but I had waited long enough and was ready to get on to the next phase.

Other costs if you have surgery are monthly office visits, *adjustments* monthly for many months if you have the Lap Band like I did, vitamins and supplements you must take religiously, protein shakes and of course, clothes that I mentioned. I will address these in the individual tips for success.

The last assumption I will mention is support from family and friends. We will talk about this in detail in my tips but if you have mixed support you *will* struggle.

I was in a relationship for five years at the time I had surgery but was with someone who liked *larger* mates and who was very thin. My partner was very unsupportive which ultimately ended our union but thankfully I had unconditional love and support from many friends, co-workers and others in my life.

At the time, my family was not nearby so they only saw photos of my progress and when I went to family holiday gatherings they were shocked at the very dramatic changes in my physical appearance.

I want to be careful that you understand very clearly that you will physically and emotionally change in dramatic ways after weight loss surgery.

These changes start immediately and the effects are constant. Your body needs to *catch up*, which doesn't always sync in rhythm and there are multiple physiological changes that occur when you lose weight this rapidly. Not all of these changes are experienced as positive in the beginning.

These psychological and emotional changes that occur can have a huge impact on your psyche. That is why it is so important that you *work out how you will balance things* and keep your life in check once you have surgery or lose a large amount of weight.

You need solid support systems in place, a stable foundation for your life and a compassionate surgical team for this to work well.

As a food addict, when people made fun of me, I usually masked my emotions by making jokes. I was 150 pounds overweight so I would say things like: *I like to live large* or laugh when people said I liked to *throw my weight around*.

I didn't have any boundaries so never understood the term *excess*. Trust me, the weight didn't come on by me *willing my mind* to gain weight. It happened as a direct result of *putting food in my mouth* - good food, bad food or any food - *it was emotional eating*.

It didn't matter about the type of emotion, either. Like any other addict, I used my addiction to *celebrate* as equally as I did to deal with my pain, boredom, stress and loneliness.

So, when I decided to have weight loss surgery, I thought I was prepared to emotionally heal my food addiction but really was *very far from knowing* what was in store for me.

I am only one person with a story to tell but I also know many others that have had different weight loss surgical procedures and I'm sure all will tell you that they were not as emotionally prepared as they could have been when they had their surgery.

It is my hope that this information will guide you as you prepare for your surgery or make other decisions to lose weight and deal with your food addiction. If you need help, there are lots of professionals to assist you.

In my individual coaching, mentoring and support groups, I am able to help others with their lives in ways that I couldn't before and someday perhaps you will be able to do the same thing.

Let's get started on how to *live large* after weight loss but do this in a balanced way. Ready, set, here we go!

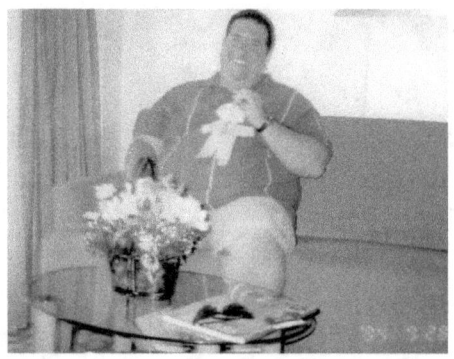

March 2008 - 330 lbs - I began a
liquid diet for 2 weeks in
preparation for
weight loss surgery

15 Tips for Success

Tip #1: Start a Journal

I tell everyone who is starting any type of new journey to write down the experience. We all have a story to tell. Some stories are more painful or glorious than others but nonetheless your story should be captured to remember.

Journaling is very powerful and allows you to look back at where you were, where you have come and also to define your challenges as well as successes. I've kept a journal at various times in my life for over thirty years since I studied abroad in college. In some of my passages, I've recalled my pain but also *many* joyful moments.

I have journaled about friendships and relationships that ran their course and was able to put my thoughts and feelings down as I started to lose weight and, now six years later, keep it off. Write everything you feel and whenever you want.

I took time each night before bed to write a paragraph in my first 90 days after surgery and then monthly afterwards but you should make this a personal experience.

In the middle of my journey, I ended a six and a half year relationship which added to my experiences but also have had many other life experiences over six years since I had surgery. Some are actually documented here in this book for the first time.

It's very important to chronicle your thoughts and feelings as well as your physical and emotional state. Not only to discuss with your medical professional but also to be able to look back a few years (which you will do) to have a better understanding of certain things that you might not have been aware of at the time.

Go get a journal if you don't already have one dedicated to weight loss - one with plenty of empty pages and start writing today!

Tip #2: Setup Your Support Network

I cannot stress this enough: If you don't have a strong, supportive network of family, friends, co-workers, professionals, etc., you will have a very long road ahead. Your support network should be challenging and push you to your limits, limits that *do* increase over time and the bar should be raised when you reach a plateau or you will stay stuck. There are plenty of times you will want to give up, that you will be in physical pain, that you will lose faith, cry, have emotional rages as your body inevitably will try to reject all the change and you *will* feel the psychological impact. Having family and friends that support this is imperative.

The same for your workplace. Your company and co-workers need to be aware of what you are doing and what this means for time away for appointments, your mental status and physical abilities to perform. This also follows accordingly for your loved ones and friends. This is very hard to do. As you won't know how your body will react to the changes in weight, you won't be able to know your emotional status. Remember this as it may be strange for you. You probably won't think you are any different. People will say: *you have changed* but this will seem like a foreign concept since the only thing you will think about is the lost weight. I assure you that your emotions and capacity to handle various situations will change.

Keep remembering your body is made up of about 60% water and the process of detoxifying your body by processing out fat will keep things constantly shifting during the weight loss process.

Make sure your closest relationships know that you might be like a *Jekyll and Hyde* for a couple of years as you go through this.

If they have questions, you might find it beneficial to meet with your medical professional or weight loss team which I think is a very good idea as some of these people need to be aware of what is going to happen after you have surgery.

A typical support network would include close family or relatives, a few true friends that can be brutally honest with you and people you work with like your boss or others you can trust to understand your emotions.

This isn't the time to rely on those you *wish or hope* will be there for you. Let those codependent thoughts leave your mind. If they aren't helpful or supportive now, they won't be as you go through this process. So, get your core support team together as soon as possible, prepare them, educate them and tell them how you will need their help to be successful.

When I had my surgery, I hoped my partner would help but thankfully I didn't plan for this and I enlisted three close friends to be there as my *go-to suppo*rt along with a very helpful co-worker who was able to assist me with any work or medical issues that arose.

My family lived out-of-state but my mother was a rock of support every week on the phone and offered me the extra financial stability I needed at various spots over the years post-surgery.

Professionally and Spiritually you might benefit from various types of counseling or group support. I had some individual therapy and ultimately went on some anti-depressant medication for a couple years after surgery on the advice of my medical professional.

I've also attended Overeaters Anonymous and other 12 Step Meetings along the way which I highly recommend for gaining a better perspective.

Many people are spiritual or religious and you might benefit from meetings at your particular faith's location with your minister or a spiritual guide. I was lucky that I had a very close person in my life that is a Life Coach and she offered support that helped me a great deal along the way. It is wonderful that I am now able to offer these types of coaching and support services after all the years of my struggling with a compulsive food addiction through my website abundantlifearchitects.com .

As I've mentioned before, these are all personal choices but having a solid support network will really help in the dark times that you will undoubtedly encounter and will also be wonderful for all your success!

Not dwelling on the dark or negative is very important as you meander through this journey. It is inevitable that you will often have challenge but staying on track and being as positive as possible will help you.

Keep remembering that you have only yourself in the end. Only *you* can keep the fire burning when you want to give up. Others will be there

to support you but it is your own willingness to

drive forward and not give up that will determine

if you will be successful long-term. You *can* do

it. You are a miracle and you are worth it!

Tip #3: Coordinate your Routine

When you make the decision to change and set the process in motion, you will need to be prepared and set up a fairly regimented daily routine with all the various things you need at your disposal that are necessary to ensure you will be successful. Every person who undertakes weight loss programs, especially weight loss surgery, will know how important routine is and consistency with eating, drinking liquids, taking supplements, etc.

It's important to get a plan together for the weeks leading up to your surgery, through the first six to eight weeks afterward and then a monthly plan going forward. The month before and two months post-surgery are vitally important to your success and set the stage for ongoing weight loss so I cannot stress enough that you must *remove all obstacles* in your path and make sure you have a set plan prior to surgery.

I do lots of Project Planning in my work and set objectives / goals that are measurable, specific and realistic - oh yeah, and one's that are *attainable.* I encourage each of you to set goals for your own routine and, in general, to set goals related to your surgery or weight loss program *as directed by your medical weight loss professionals.*

In my particular case, I was paying for the surgery, so I had set some pretty aggressive goals for myself in the first year which I will talk about later. As a beginning step, you should write down all the things that are needed to get you set up for success. Here are some of my suggestions that I used as part of my planning which might help you in your preparations:

Get a food processor for your Protein Shakes and other foods (I recommend the Magic Bullet as these are compact, easy to use and make a perfect shake with some ice).

There are lots of variations of mini food processors and juicers on the market so you will want to choose what works best for you.

You will need something as eventually even the best of us get tired of the same thing for months on end and need something to change up the routine. The Magic Bullet is easy to use and to clean. It also has cups that attach so you can sip right from your creation!

Buy small 4 oz plastic food containers, several 20 oz plastic shakers and a large pill dispenser for one week supplies of vitamins.

Be aware that after weight loss surgery, your food portions will most likely be no more than two ounces as a rule of thumb. Therefore, you will need lots of *small* containers for any food. I still use these and they help very much for *portion-controlled size*s.

The 20 oz shakers are like a best friend as you will probably be having three to four 35 g protein shakes a day for at least the first year.

Personally, I just wanted to get my protein shakes down so I made mine with only about six to eight ounces of water (combined with 1 ½ scoops of whey stack protein powder) to get the 35g of protein in each shake.

Everyone is different. The more time you have and the more elaborate or creative that you want to be is up to you. That's why the Magic Bullet is great because you can mix lots of things in with like fruit, vegetables and even all your daily vitamins and supplements like I did for a long time!

Regarding vitamins and supplements, since you will be taking vitamins from A to Z on a daily basis, I suggest you buy a large pill dispenser that will hold about twenty different types of vitamins and supplements.

Mine looked like a mini-suitcase with a snap lock that I bought at GNC for a low cost. I was able to put at least a two week supply of most vitamins and supplements in this container which really helped me to organize my routine for taking my vitamins.

You need to be organized about taking your vitamins and supplements to avoid medical issues with energy, hair loss, bone density issues, depression, etc. Your physician and weight loss clinic will be the experts on what vitamins and supplements to take for your weight loss procedure and you *need to follow their instructions to the lette*r. If you don't, your body will let you know.

In my case, I developed a Vitamin D deficiency. I had to have a special injection and then be monitored for several months when this was discovered. I strongly encourage you not to fool around with your vitamin and supplement routine as it is critical to your overall success.

Taking vitamins and supplements is part of your daily routine and having the proper container for these will make it much easier for you.

Buy a good scale to weigh yourself if you don't already have one. If you are like me when I weighed myself at 330 pounds, the last things I wanted to do was get on the scale and most standard home scales don't go past 300 pounds so I didn't have a functional scale until I bought one right before my surgery. I actually got a very cool Weight Watchers Digital Scale that gave other good information about BMI (Body Mass Index), water levels and bone density. I recommend you consider these to keep track of your progress on a weekly basis.

You probably will go to your particular weight loss clinic monthly but it will be beneficial if you check your weight *weekly* as well. Please *do not look at your weight daily* or worry about whether you are wearing clothes or shoes, etc. when you weigh as this is unimportant.

Try to weigh yourself at the same time on the same day each week after you shower and then make sure to record this in your journal along with all the other percentages (if any) on your digital scale.

Doing anything else is doomed for problems *as your weight fluctuates daily.* Your body will be processing fat out at lightning speeds and it doesn't always calibrate like you want simply because it's your weigh in day at the doctor's office or the time you step on the scale at home.

Later in Tip # 10 we will talk about plateaus and stalling out on your weight loss whi*ch will happen several times along your journey* so be patient. Having a scale is not to make you dependent on it, rather, to monitor progress and to maintain a level of accountability.

Determine what type of Protein Shakes, Vitamins and Supplements you will use. In Tip # 6, I describe this in detail but you will need to have all of the recommended items ready to go the day you start your pre-surgery liquid diet or whenever you start your vitamin and supplement program as directed by your physician or weight loss program.

In the pre-surgery phase, there are also some folks who may prefer pre-made protein shakes and others that like powdered protein. All protein shakes are different. I am speaking only about my particular program at the St. Francis Weight Loss Center. This program was highly successful for several thousand people over several years, however, you should consult *your individual program and follow their particular guidelines.*

Whatever you decide to do with protein after weight loss surgery, it needs to be consistent and follow the same daily routine.

Keep the little 1 ounce cups they will give you at the hospital post-surgery for sipping liquid. If you have weight loss surgery, during recovery and throughout your stay at the hospital, you will be on liquid for the entire time.

You will be given 1oz cups that are used for taking medicine and are used for you to sip fluids after your surgical procedure. This most likely will be water and / or apple juice but remember is to save these tiny plastic cups as they will help you for the first couple of month with portions that you can tolerate as, initially, these will only be liquids.

It might seem crazy but I left the hospital after 24 hours with about 100 of these little gems and I still have a handful six years after my procedure. Why? *Convenience.*

You will no longer be able to gulp down water with vitamins, you will be on a liquid diet for several weeks after surgery and you will really find having these measuring cups handy when you need to sip, so I encourage you to stock up since they will toss them if not! Something else worth mentioning, you will feel unwell after surgery and be groggy.

Even if you feel too ill to sip or don't want to take in liquids, it is important that you get as much fluid down as you can. You will need to be very hydrated in the days, weeks, months and for *years* to come!

Make sure your Finances are in order. This is really important. Nothing will derail your happiness than if you encounter financial issues along the way.

For me, I knew I had to pre-pay the surgeons and hospital as a package two weeks before I could be admitted. I also knew I had to pay about $60-$75 a month for Protein Shakes, Vitamins and Supplements as well as a $150 a month fee for my Lap Band Adjustments.

If you have Lap Band Surgery, each month you need it tightened (or adjusted) to make it work properly and this starts a whole new process that goes on for about 2 years to get the right amount of *fill* (saline that is injected into a port that tightens or loosens the band around your stomach).

If your insurance isn't paying, you need to be sure you can afford these monthly visits as these are vital to your success. You really need to be financially stable so you know there are no financial surprises that would trigger you, as a food addict, to try to cheat or eat things that will make you ill. Financial problems can sabotage or derail your weight loss goals. It does happen. Life, that is.

We cannot plan for everything even though we might want to hold on to that control as addicts. In losing weight, you will have to give up a good amount of control to actually start taking control of your life again and financial stability is part of this in the overall life balance.

As part of your overall *physical* change in losing weight, you will need to buy new clothes several times throughout the weight loss process and this costs money as well.

There are many creative solutions to replacing your wardrobe a few times a year for about two years that are cost-effective.

If you ever thought of donating to charity, this is the time! You will save vast amounts of money buying your clothes at places like the Goodwill, Value Village, Salvation Army or the local bargain basement and you will actually have fun in the process!

You should be prepared financially as this is a cost for about every 50 pounds depending on your body shape and size.

Looking back, I don't know what I was thinking when I decided to buy a house three months after surgery! It was, perhaps, one of the most risky things I could have done and a major life stressor that I added to my challenging work, relationship and daily weight loss regimen. Make sure you are ready for the unexpected as your mind is going to do some very creative things as the pounds start to come off.

Work schedule. Most of you will have work to return to if you have surgery or even if you don't have surgery, you will have a life that includes some sort of work routine on a daily basis that will change for sure if you have weight loss surgery.

If you have a desk job, returning to work is actually not too bad as most of these surgical procedures are now Laparoscopic and you are usually back to work in a week or two at the outside. *Please make sure to take the full amount of time as prescribed by your surgeon's recommendation* without faltering.

It is a matter of life or death in some instances and I won't pretend to know anyone's individual circumstances but just know that even though you may not look like much has happened on the outside (at first), your body has just endured a major procedure and needs to properly heal and not be rushed in this process.

Do not and I repeat ***do no*t** *try to do anything outside of the routine that your physician or weight loss center has authorized.*

This includes lifting, straining yourself, sitting or lying in positions that are not recommended and, especially at work, staying in the same position without moving. Your doctor will let you know the rules and I am mentioning it here in the work routine because if you don't follow the rules, you will end up missing work and this can result in other complications.

You must inform your employer of what you are doing as well as your co-workers. You should ask them all for their support.

If you don't have the support of your employer, you can still proceed but it might be difficult if your company doesn't offer a Leave of Absence or Short Term Disability Plan It is important to sit down with them in advance and set clear expectations about what you will need to be successful at work post-surgery.

At minimum, it is making sure you have the time off work that you will need for the surgery, for the monthly (or more frequent) visits to the doctor, support groups, other specialists, etc.

Most employers will be very happy to hear of your weight loss surgery plans because if you are considerably overweight, most likely you have had lots of other weight-related issues that have had you at the doctor.

Informing them of upcoming Lap Band surgery helps them to know that you are taking responsibility for your life and ensures that they are aware you are serious about getting your health issues resolved for good.

Sometimes it's more than just time-off work. Many employers have unwritten expectations for you and won't always understand when you need to take care of yourself, physically or emotionally, when there are deadlines. Be careful when you select the date you have surgery. I decided to have mine right around April as this was a good time of year with the business I worked in at the time.

Whatever you decide, make sure you have properly scheduled your work life and personal life to be in balance to be as focused as possible on your weight loss program.

The last thing I will mention is the impact of food in the workplace. We've all worked where nearby there are many fast food spots nearby and folks all chip in for lunch orders. There are also the birthday parties and work potlucks that don't stop just because you had weight loss surgery. I had both the blessing and the curse to work with nurses for most of my career. They are fantastic cooks!

I've learned the best recipes and tasted incredible food at the work buffets over the years but with a serious weight loss program this all changes.

If you have weight loss surgery, some of these foods are impossible to eat as your body will no longer tolerate the food. If you can eat them, most of the preparations might not be the healthy choice for you so beware.

As everyone knew I had surgery, it made it easy to decline the food and I just brought my own little containers and ate my own snacks with a smile on my face knowing I had eaten it all before and I was making a life change. Believe me, after awhile you won't even notice and you *may* try the occasional chip, dip or whatever is at the buffet.

Remember that your mind doesn't change just because you had surgery or have lost weight. *You are still a food addict.* You might not have incredible cravings for all foods but the thought of certain foods will never leave your mind and can still trigger emotional eating. You have to conquer all of this to stay balanced as you progress.

Clear out the Cupboards. I know, you somehow may think the Oreo's and Nacho Doritos will be fine to keep around with the Ruffles Sour Cream and the Twinkies since *you* can't eat them anymore, right? Wrong!

You *can and will try* so do yourself a huge favor now and *rid yourself of any and all bad foods that are lurking in your fridge , freezer or cupboards*!

Take your food to a food pantry as a donation if needed or give it to friends, family and coworkers. In my situation, and you might have this, too, I had the painful issue that my partner loved eating junk food. To solve this dilemma, we agreed on specific cabinets and I had ones dedicated to me as well as specific areas of the fridge and freezer.

Since most of my meals were liquid in the beginning it, wasn't too much of an issue but as I progressed to solid food after about three months, it was good that I set this up before surgery and if you have a family, this will be an ongoing challenge as you are probably the caretaker and meal-maker. You will constantly have to interact with foods you don't (or can't) eat.

I didn't say shouldn't, I said *can*'t for a reason as your body won't tolerate these foods and you will be sick or really feel discomfort. It's a good rule to start everyone on a healthy living routine from the start . If you have the love and support of your family (which is absolutely necessary for success), this shouldn't be an issue.

If you don't, you will need guidance from your medical professional, a support group or a mentor / life coach that can provide other suggestions.

Tip #4: Start An Exercise Program

Your doctor or weight loss center will instruct you on when it is safe to begin exercise or for any type of activity post-surgery. It's very important that if you are considering surgery you start getting active now (pre-surgery or weight loss) and not wait.

For most of us who allowed the pounds to come on over the years and make excuses why we couldn't lead a more active lifestyle, you will not get sympathy from me.

I spent *years* living sedately and eventually my biggest walk was to the refrigerator from my upstairs bedroom!

When I weighed 330 pounds, I was at a Christmas Eve party and started talking to a friend I knew who was a personal trainer. I had used a couple personal trainers in the past and they were very good but my mindset was not focused on using exercise as a tool to manage my weight.

To be honest, I don't *love* exercise like some folks. I don't look forward to a day at the gym nor do I crave working. I wish I had a better story to tell you that I did but I don't. Am I much more active today? Absolutely. Can I do many things I couldn't before surgery? Yes.

I think you have to determine what is right for you and know that your thoughts and feelings about the gym, exercising and becoming more active all will change very much over time.

I started telling my friend that I wanted to have weight loss surgery in about three months and asked if could help me to get more physically fit before my surgery.

It's always nice to have someone else to work out with in these situation so, as luck would have it, I had another friend that wasn't actually overweight but he wanted to get in better shape.

We started working out 3 times a week in the small gym in the building where I lived. I encourage you to find someplace that fits your personality and will allow you to feel OK.

We've all spent too many years feeling ashamed of our bodies - especially at places that people go to look pretty and strut around.

I'm sure you know the pain that results from being overweight and walking on the treadmill at the gym. I knew what they were not thinking: *wow, isn't that great? That obese man is doing something to help save his life.*

I felt they were saying something more along the lines of: *Look at that fat guy! What the hell is he taking up space on the treadmill when he's just going to stop by Wendy's after he works out!*

Maybe you don't feel like this but I sure did. Having a gym in my building worked very well as there usually were no others around and privacy was great.

You might not be able to afford a personal trainer but there are so many free or low cost web applications out now that can help. I actually bartered with my trainer for other personal coaching services and since my friend split the cost with me (at the gym which was an amenity of my building), it was cost-effective.

Make sure you have a place you like, that you know you can go to that meets your needs for space and privacy as you start out. It's very important.

The other thing you should do is find others that work out, walk, run, boat, cycle etc. to mentor you along your exercise routine. Almost always this is free or perhaps in exchange for a nice meal or a drink for their help.

This is actually pretty easy as there will be lots of very fit friends you know that you can easily tap into as resources and *most of them will love to talk about their healthy lives, exercise routines* and almost all I found are willing to be part of *your* program if you ask.

I had a friend who loved to go walking. She was incredibly fit and could run circles around me but she pushed me and encouraged me to work harder and faster and when I thought I was done walking or running she insisted we do another lap! After months walking with her on summer nights around Green Lake (just outside of Seattle), I started to enjoy the feeling of staying active not because I had to but as I wanted to do various activities.

I realize not all of you live in climates that allow outdoor activities year round but getting out in nature and walking around is great for your mental health as well as your physical well-being. Why not start an exercise or more active lifestyle routine now if you haven't already?

Make sure your doctor or healthcare professional says you are healthy and can start an exercise program but then by all means - get moving!

A little caveat - there *will* come a time when in the weight loss process *you might be losing too much weight* each month and you may need to slow down your exercise routine or your weight loss is stalled and you need to increase your routine.

Hard to believe but it's true and I experienced both a couple of times in the first two years after surgery.

I had my Lap Band adjusted too tight initially and was working out with a trainer and started losing 17 to 20 pounds per month, which was too much for my healthy, gradual weight loss.

So, I just walked and stopped weight training to allow my body to catch up with the adjustments. I also opened my Lap Band to allow for more food intake so I didn't lose as much weight.

These are all decisions you will make working with *your* team of professionals so just be flexible and open to the change. You need this flexibility with your exercise routine to stay balanced and healthy as you progress.

Tip #5: The Liquid Diet

A liquid protein diet will soon become a major part of your life for at least two years if you plan to be successful after weight loss surgery. I've said that this process is a journey, well, enjoying your liquid diet of protein shakes, clear broth and other liquids like water and soups are part of this life if you decide to have surgery.

Even if you don't have surgery, the cleansing properties of having a liquid fast for a couple of days each month can actually be quite good.

Your surgeon and weight loss program will have a set process or program for you to follow that usually begins at least two weeks before your surgery and continues for about six to eight weeks after you have surgery.

Yes, if you do the math you most likely won't have any solid foods for about 8-12 weeks before and after surgery. Even then, you first introduce soft and easy to digest foods so plan that your life is going to be very different.

Many weight loss programs recommend three Protein Shakes a day that will provide about 100 grams of protein each day, 64 ounces of water and will allow you to have broth or sugar-free jello as part of your liquid program. These vary but it's important that you get used to this as a new part of life and embrace the shift from solid to liquid for the first few months after surgery.

I remember when I had to start my liquid diet all too well. I was on a family vacation and we were on a cruise that sailed out of Ft. Lauderdale, Florida. On the morning we docked, there was food in the main dining areas but nothing I could eat. I could only drink protein shakes and clear liquid broth along with a vast assortment of vitamins and supplements that I barely could pronounce at the time.

Let me be honest with you, plan to tell folks that you will be an absolute tyrant when you first start on a liquid diet in preparation for weight loss surgery!

I was really angry when I stopped having food and furious that I couldn't eat solid food even though I knew I had to do this for medical reasons to shrink my liver and the fat surrounding it in order to avoid surgical complications. It didn't matter when everyone was eating pancakes and bacon and with juices and pastries.

I gulped down my first protein shake and was so unsatisfied but knew I needed to start somewhere. Thus my world was forever changed: no solid food and 3 Protein Shakes a day. Yowza.

I learned to love liquids and broth. To this day, my first food choice is soup. I've become very accustomed to sipping on liquids as my first choice for food. I still eat soft foods over six years later by choice as my body won't tolerate certain foods with my Lap Band.

Protein Shakes, Water, Broth and Sugar Free Jello are not bad and keep it real when you are making life changes and better food choices.

Eventually you will choose whether you decide to go back to old patterns and old ways of behaving rather than staying the course on your weight loss journey.

I guarantee you won't be drinking shakes forever and eventually will wean yourself from most of the things you did in your first two years but you must be diligent in balancing your food intake as it is the key to keeping your food addiction under control and staying at a healthy weight.

Tip #6: Protein, Water and Vitamins

When I was in my pre-surgery nutrition class about one month before my procedure, there was a woman who had the Gastric Bypass surgery eight years prior who worked with the weight loss clinic's nutritionist and she was extremely helpful since I was completely clueless about the diet after surgery.

She told our class of about 35 people that this is a life-altering procedure and that our bodies would no longer eat or process food the same way ever again.

She showed us different Protein Shake options (the one *she* liked was actually not the one I eventually chose), talked about the process from pre-surgery to three months after and beyond.

What sticks in my mind most about this four hour class were her words at the conclusion of our session: *Remember this if you don't remember anything else from the class. Have your 3 protein shakes, your water, your vitamins and supplements and then whatever food you can get down.*

I'm also remembering the woman who asked in the class if she could still eat popcorn after the surgery. Another woman (who was having a *second* surgery as she gained all her original weight back after the first procedure) replied, *honey, let me tell you, the last* *thing you're gonna want afte*r weight *loss*

surgery is popcorn!

It was actually about three years after surgery that I started eating popcorn. Not that it's bad per se or that I couldn't eat it but *you will start to make choices of what you ea*t and what types of food will nourish your body versus those that will just simply continue to feed your addiction and provide empty calories.

You first must decide what Protein Shake, Vitamins and Supplements you will use. This step is crucial. Your doctor will have a regimen and program as well as recommend several local suppliers.

Think of this step as *one of your most important* as it is going to determine about 75% of what you will be having as your *food* for at least the first year.

I could write volumes on this topic but will leave this to you to sort out with your individual program but will offer some recommendations of course.

Not all Protein Shakes are alike. There are literally hundreds of types, flavors and tastes. The same goes for Vitamins and Supplements. You will want to choose a good Whey Stack Protein Shake that tastes good when blended with water.

This isn't a trip to the Dairy Queen or your favorite Ice-Cream spot for a shake and you will be using these to basically get all your essential protein and other key nutrients in your diet as you won't be able to get this through food.

I was very lucky as my particular weight loss clinic had two folks that had the procedure ten years prior and started a company selling (and shipping) protein shakes, vitamins and supplement called The Vitalady. I went to their office which and tasted about 30 different types of protein shakes from Cookies and Creme to Banana.

There were so many amazing shakes! I encourage you to explore your options and not to just go to an expensive brand nutrition store. I did this initially and spent about triple what I now spend at The Vitalady and get free shipping with my order.

I still purchase all my shakes, vitamins and supplements from the Vitalady and what I like about this type of grass roots company is that all their products are great and these folks understand your situation. They have had weight loss surgery and *know exactly what you need for any type of surgery*. They can really guide you.

I knew absolutely nothing other than what I was told to buy from my weight loss program and I was so confused.

There are liquid vitamins, sublingual, chewable and standard types. Since you will initially be taking about 20+ vitamins and supplements daily, I hope you investigate what you like and how these taste as this is very important to your routine.

For me, I wanted *easy* and the liquid vitamins were too expensive, so I chose to get as many sublingual and chewable *flavored* vitamins and supplements as humanly possible.

Taste, you will soon learn, takes on an entirely new meaning when most of your daily meals are protein shakes with vitamins and supplements!

I tried several different varieties of protein shakes. Since I travelled for work and it is almost impossible to travel with a blender and everything you need, the Vitalady had pre-packaged *portions* of various types of shakes that could be taken on the road and easily poured into a shaker.

You can also pre-measure portions you need for your trip and put these in a gallon sized Ziplock bag with a scoop to measure for your shaker. Add water and shake!

In the end, you will find your own routine about taking vitamins and supplements but you must take them daily without fail!

Your doctor will give you very good details on what can be taken together as some vitamins and supplements cannot due to the way they counteract in the absorption process but any nutritionist or weight loss clinic can provide you with this important information.

I didn't talk too much about water but you will discuss this with the weight loss program as part of your diet. Most programs recommend 64 ounces of water a day (8 glasses) but this can vary by person, so make sure you know what you need to stay hydrated.

Remember, your body is comprised of about 60% water. Think of yourself like a car and that needs water to run properly or the engine will overheat.

Your body is exactly the same. It needs water (fluids) to process out all the fat and toxins that will be part of your weight loss journey. In order to stay focused, balanced and feeling well, you need to keep these levels well-regulated.

Personally, I am not the type of person that loves to walk around with my water bottle with the spout and sip all day.

I also get bored with plain water at times. For me, I like lemonade and various flavors which today are in abundance with the squirt bottles with concentrated juice flavors and also the traditional single-serve powders.

Whatever you choose, it is important that you like the taste and that it is refreshing. I love chilled water so it's fantastic to have my Brita filtered water in my fridge and when I am on the go I often take along one of my 20 oz shakers with water.

You will need to talk to your doctor about drinking coffee, tea, sodas and of course alcohol. You also should be aware of the effects that sodium, sugar, caffeine and alcohol have on your body.

You need to stay hydrated at all times to keep your body processing fat and toxins. Sodium, caffeine, alcohol and most all processed foods don't work in harmony with this process and can slow down or stall your progress.

It is very important to your successful weight loss goals that the body keep processing like a well-oiled machine. The liquid diet is part of this and needed in order yourself balanced at all times.

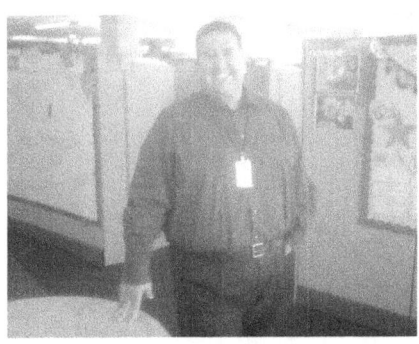

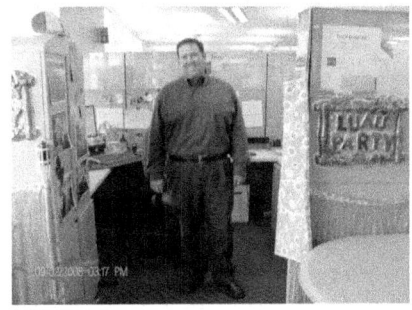

Photos of me *in transition* at 3 months and 9 months after weight loss surgery.

Tip #7: Food Intake and Cravings

From time-to-time, we all have a craving for something. Some people crave sugar and sweets, some like salty snacks, others enjoy dairy products and many desire *all* the above!

As your journey progresses, so will your cravings change as will the types and amounts of food you choose to put in your body.

I remember someone telling me one time years ago that *my body was a temple* and I needed to treat it as such only putting food and nutrients in it that would let it know how much I appreciated it.

Well, that may be true but when I was at the height of my food active addiction, I assure you that I thought Dunkin' Donuts, Burger King Whoppers and Papa John's Pepperoni Pizza *was* celebrating my body!

We all know the damage our addictions have done to our bodies and the pain that we have endured being food addicts. I'm not going to focus on something you already know, rather, I am wanting to make sure you are very prepared before you have surgery or go on any type of extreme weight loss program that you are know what you can eat. This also includes foods you can tolerate, how your body reacts to food and especially how you will deal with your new body.

In the past, you have made bad food choices and it's important to know what to do when your system tries to get mad at you for making new, healthy choices.

Weight loss is only one piece of the puzzle when it comes to eating and food cravings. Most likely you, like me, are an emotional eater and this is what can paralyze a food addict and keep you held back from your long-term success.

Understanding the emotional aspects behind why you are eating is the key to looking at your food intake and cravings in a different, more healthy perspective.

I will continue to refer to what I said in Tip #6: have your 3 protein shakes each day and 4 if you get cravings, take your daily vitamins/supplements, drink your required fluids. Then whatever food you can get down.

When you have your 35g servings of Whey Stack Protein three times a day you are getting over 100 grams of solid protein which will keep you from craving lots of bad foods that are not on your approved list post-surgery. I will talk more about some major no no's in Tip # 9.

After about eight weeks on a liquid diet and pretty much thereafter, your body will be used to this protein source and cravings for your past will seem to melt away as quickly as the pounds start to drop off.

The multitude of vitamins and supplements you will be taking religiously along with your protein shakes will be giving you the required nutrients you need to supplement for the lack of actual food intake.

I will say this again because I want to be very clear that *IT IS EXTREMELY IMPORTANT BEFORE YOU START ANY TYPE OF WEIGHT LOSS PROGRAM THAT YOU SPEAK WITH A MEDICAL PROFESSIONAL.*

It is required as part of any surgical procedure and each procedure has different pros and cons but also has some variations on what you can eat and drink.

Folks that have the Gastric Bypass, for example, must take some additional supplements as their food absorption process is different than that of someone who has the Lap Band like I did.

Please check with your medical weight loss program and follow their directions *to the letter* regarding what they require for protein intake, vitamins and supplements.

If you're similar to me, though, you will want to *test* the process. After I got home from the hospital, about a week later I had a craving for food. It was like a starchy carb craving and guess what? Yep, I just happened to see some macaroni salad in the fridge and it was calling my name.

I knew the doctor said *no solid food*, especially no pasta. I knew I had not had any solid food in my system now for about a month but I tempted like I was in the Garden of Eden. I took a small teaspoon and ate it. It wasn't 15 seconds before I threw up! It hurt, oh did it hurt! My body was not able to tolerate any food since for the past month only liquid had gone through.

I hate to admit this but I did try to test myself to see what would happen on a few occasions and it was always the same result: I would feel very nauseous, uncomfortable and within minutes, I would throw up.

Even to this day if I eat something I know my body doesn't tolerate (and I want to check in and see as if by some miracle it will be different), I get sick.

I'm not going to spend lots of time telling you what you can and cannot eat as this is best left to your supervised weight loss program, the nutritionist and, well, your body. Each diet and exercise plan is different and so is your body. What one person can eat, another cannot. Also, what they say you can eat is not always what you can or *if* you can, it can take hours to digest making you feel really uncomfortable.

I had the Lap Band surgery and have a small band at the top portion of my stomach that was adjusted monthly for almost two years. As it was adjusted, the opening from the top portion of my stomach got smaller so it took longer for food to process into my stomach.

Basically, after any weight loss surgery, think of your stomach as about the size of an egg. Whatever an egg can hold is what your stomach can and that's not very much. Why I chose the Lap Band is that it is *restrictive for food intake* and since I was a food addict who loved eating, I knew that if I was careful and ate the correct foods I would be able to keep my weight off and not regain.

Ultimately I had lost too much weight and after my skin removal surgery, I had to open my Lap Band to allow more food intake. My particular Lap Band was also at 11.2 cc of fluid (most standard Lap Bands can hold up to 15 cc of fluid) which was very restrictive to the point I could not hold down water or my protein shakes so I needed to take immediate corrective action to avoid health complications.

I am now at a very comfortable 7.5 cc of fluid and can eat and drink but it still can take hours to digest things I don't eat very often, like meat or raw vegetables. So, I try to avoid eating the things I know just don't work and eating soft foods or liquids to give me my nutrients without lots of extra supplementation.

You will need to find a healthy balance for yourself. You must be patient as it takes time. It took me over three years to get my Lap Band adjusted to the correct level after I had skin removal surgery as it was too tight and I looked unhealthy at the weight I was at which was 25 pounds *less than* my original goal weight.

Even now, I cannot eat any type of eggs, most raw vegetables, bread, heavy foods like meat, certain fruits and basically things that take time to digest in your system. These food items remain stuck in the top portion of my stomach (called the *pouch*) before going through the Lap Band to my actual stomach and soon thereafter I start to feel nauseated and then it's all downhill from there.

Everyone will have their own reactions to food, regardless of the type of weight loss surgical procedure. You will only know by trying a certain food, seeing if it works and if it doesn't try again at different times or after several months (or years). It's all about a balancing what works and doesn't work after you have weight loss surgery.

Your body has no idea what it is processing from an actual food type or texture point-of-view. All it knows is that certain types of foods will enter into the body for processing. The body then reacts accordingly by sending enzymes to help in the digestion process.

How it all works, I will leave to the experts but I know enough to tell you that your body *is* a temple when it comes to food intake after you have any type of weight loss surgery or program. What you put in to it *will* have an immediate impact on how you feel.

Remember this when you even *think* about diving into that Late Night Chili Cheese Dog when you are lamenting: *Why did I do this? Why did I have this surgery?* How do I know? Yeah, you already know how I know because that was me about six months after weight loss surgery!

The end result of your emotional outburst will make you sick almost instantly because *food can no longer be used as your addiction.* Your surgery created a wall that, even if you try to break through, I guarantee your misery is not worth it.

The rewards, however, are incredible if you stick to your weight loss plan, follow the rules, heal your mind, body and spirit *and* don't intentionally sabotage your success.

The food choices you will make will be what will comprise the *fuel* for your body to properly function and, with practice, patience and support from others, you will find that you will be eating tiny portions of healthy foods that you can tolerate.

Remember those 3-4 ounce plastic containers? Use these and you will be having nutritious and filling food portions probably within three to six months and, after about a year, you will be eating actual meals.

These will be much smaller portions but by this time food portion control will be part of your daily routine just like taking your vitamins and supplements.

Remember that *balance will become the success factor* on your weight loss journey. The word balance *must* become your barometer for everything you now do in life. You *will* find ways to *cheat* after surgery and that is normal.

It's a reality you need to be aware of and I discuss this in Tip #13. If you don't follow your weight loss plan, *you really are only hurting yourself* in the end and letting your emotional addiction to food control your life.

Please stay the course! It's worth it and *YOU*
are worth it!

Tip #8: Food Intolerance

I've talked about food intake and also have
mentioned food intolerance that often occurs
with folks that have weight loss surgery. For the
standard person who is dieting and working out,
yes, you might not like all the foods you are
eating but to the individual that has had weight
loss surgery, this takes on an entirely new
meaning.

Basically, you are going from *living to eat* as a
food addict to *eating to live* as someone post
weight loss surgery. There are several types of
weight loss surgery so be careful that you follow

the strict guidelines of your particular program because they do vary.

Your particular weight loss program is there for you. They will answer any medical questions and concerns you have at any time. This is especially true for food intolerance.

It is inevitable that your body will reject almost everything you try to ingest that is not a healthy food choice in the beginning of your weight loss program and most assuredly for years after weight loss surgery.

Sometimes this can occur instantly, other times you will feel like you just had a huge holiday meal in two bites. On many occasions, you can get very nauseated and ultimately find yourself sprinting to a restroom. The worst type of food intolerance, though, will be the foods that seem to just sit and wait forever to pass through the Lap Band or seem to linger for hours before they fully digest.

Planning for food intolerance is part of your new life after weight loss surgery. You can attempt to plan things by avoiding eating establishments, eating anything that isn't on your approved list of foods or by saying no when solicited to eat something you know will make you ill.

This is all nice to write but this is the real world and you have a life to live. You are also a food addict like me and probably will push the limits to see what you can tolerate any time, any place or anywhere you happen to find a food you like (or a food your brain is telling you that you need to satisfy an emotional need).

It is important that you *always have an exit that is available* in case of an emergency when you indulge and the food is not tolerated. Sit on the outside of the restaurant booth, in a chair you can easily excuse yourself at an event, on the aisle at the movie theatre and have a disposable bag handy when you travel in the car.

I have had several times I needed to used the air-sickness bag on airplanes or had to pull over on the side of the road as I was ill. You do not need to be embarrassed or the hero anymore. Don't be ashamed as this happens. It should not by any means occur once you understand what you can, and cannot, eat.

Once you understand your body and reaction to various foods (and portions), you will be fine. If you are having any issues, please speak to your weight loss program to avoid complications and in very serious situations, an eating disorder.

After you have Lap Band surgery, you that you can sip liquid up to the point of eating food but then must stop all liquid for about 1 hour to let your food pass through the band.

They also say not to *bolt* your food, *chug* down liquids, *avoid* soda or *fizzy* drinks and *spicy* foods. Tell a food addict not to bolt their food down? it's a learning process! I did everything I *wasn't* supposed to do in the beginning and, of course, was ill too many times to mention. I think why they say to avoid spicy food and carbonated beverages is that these don't feel good when they are coming back up after food intolerance.

If you bolt your food, regardless of food tolerance, you *will* be sick. The same goes with drinking fluids, so don't guzzle down your protein shakes. If you drink something too quickly, you probably will be sick.

If you have the Lap Band surgery, after your first bite of food wait before having liquids or I guarantee you will be sick. There is nothing worse than your body getting nauseous and you feeling dizzy and then needing to run to a bathroom or anyplace you can find to throw up.

Your friends, family and co-workers should understand your food tolerance issues so they are aware why you need to sometimes excuse yourself a few times during a meal.

This is not medically proven but I personally determined that tapping my chest just above the Lap Band helped the discomfort. Some people asked if I was having a heart-attack or choking which wasn't good, so be cautious if you try this approach.

I did find that standing up and walking a bit was the most successful in these situations. As awkward as it seems, I had to let folks know that drinking water didn't *help* food go down, it made the feeling worse. I explained this like a clogged drain.

Putting water on top of the clog only creates more liquid blockage. Foods like bread, rice, pasta all expand with liquid and *block the drain* so be cautious when eating these foods. If you choose to, do so at your own risk and have your exit nearby!

It's important you realize that you are shifting your entire lifestyle. Most people in the United States are constantly on the go, rushing to and fro and eating their meals in a hurried frenzy. *Stop that pattern*!

If you don't have surgery, it's time to slow down so you can take time to enjoy your food, to savour it and to actually think about what you are putting into your body.

I wish I could tell you I did this all the time but I didn't. I am a food addict and it has taken years of practice to set mealtimes and follow a routine. Usually when I rush, I am stressed. When you are stressed, your body gets tense and when you tense all your internal organs and muscles contract making normal digestion virtually impossible.

If you have a Lap Band or have had another type of weight loss procedure, if you are rushed or stressed, it will be almost impossible to eat or to tolerate your food.

Think of stress even *without* surgery. When you are stressed, how often do you really want to eat? You are too worked up or busy. I never found myself driving to Denny's for sliders and onion rings in the middle of an argument nor did I want to gulp down a Protein Shake *after* I had weight loss surgery.

You *internalize* your stress and want to self-soothe at a later, more relaxing time.

That's when your food addiction is most insidious and creative. You are at home, nibbling or eating in private. You stop off for a pie on your way home from work or a fast food location drive through. The dilemma you will experience after weight loss surgery is that you won't be able to self-soothe much as your stomach is the size of an egg!

Prepare for alternatives to stress reduction in healthier ways like a walk, going to the gym, doing a hobby you like or volunteer work to help others.

To avoid food intolerance issues, make a *plan* for your meals and have them all set for what you will be doing at the time. If you are traveling, bring your shakers and protein mix so you know you are getting your 3 shakes as you most likely won't be able to eat anything at the hotel breakfast buffet.

You also won't be able to eat full meals any longer like you did before weight loss surgery. You will need to be upfront with co-workers, family and the restaurant you go to that you have have had surgery and you cannot eat certain things due to food intolerances. I will talk much more about this in Tip # 11 about new ways to cope.

If you have weight loss surgery (and even if you do not), life is about balance and the careful art of being able to satisfy your needs while at the same time being able to stay focused and follow a plan. If you will allow yourself the time to get used to your new body, its new rhythm and the changes it is undergoing, you will be very pleased with the outcome.

Tip #9: The No-No list

Your weight loss program or medical professional will give you the list of things that you cannot eat or drink after you have weight loss surgery. It will come as no surprise that this list will be similar to most diets you have been on before.

Let's all be honest with ourselves that we could all write a book on our failed attempts, broken promises and heartaches from eating foods that comfort us but leave us empty in the end. The thing that hurt me after having weight loss surgery was something I loved (food) was taken away from me.

Food comforted me, food was there when everyone and everything in my life seemed to be awful. If you are like me, you will mourn the loss of some of your best *food* friends like bread, rice, pasta and sugar. Trust me, though, they don't leave forever, they get replaced by different foods and different ways to cope with the way your brain reacts to your emotional eating habits.

Restriction has its limits and does not prevent you from your addiction. Therefore, you must follow your weight loss plan and recommendations from your weight loss program, physician and/or registered dietician.

When I took the required nutrition class before my surgery, they went over many things but I remembered the list that was written down for everyone having any type of weight loss surgery: NO BREAD, RICE, PASTA, MILK, SUGAR, CAFFEINE, JUICE.

I didn't understand Milk at first but it was explained to me that Milk has some type of chemical that reacts in your body and can cause you to get hungry. I am not sure if this has been medically proven but I wasn't a milk lover anyway so this wasn't a big deal.

My plan allowed me dairy products (but not Milk), which I still don't quite understand. I like cheese and other dairy products and was happy I did not have any dairy or lactose intolerance.

Years before, I actually stopped *juicing* when I learned how much sugar is in just a small glass so this also wasn't an issue. Bread, rice, pasta were difficult to say farewell to after weight loss surgery. I loved all of these foods and yes, I now eat some of these in tiny portions but it took me several years to reintroduce these in my diet.

After weight loss surgery, the way food digests will change and starchy carbohydrates are difficult for some folks, like me, to digest.

Caffeine may also a No-No on some weight loss plans. Although I lived in Seattle at the time, I wasn't a coffee drinker nor did I drink much tea, so I didn't feel like I was giving anything up.

There are many *coffee's (and I use this term loosely)* from these gourmet coffee houses which can add a couple thousand calories a day to your diet if you are not careful due to their sugar content. They will derail your success as these liquids will go down and usually process fairly easily, especially warm beverages.

If you have a Gastric Bypass surgical procedure, prepare for dumping syndrome which I have been told is an absolute nightmare. I really like soda. With all the *zero and ten calorie beverages* and, even caffeine free zero and ten beverages, these might seem tempting.

You should be aware of the sodium content in these beverages and even though I like these, I try to limit my intake and choose water as much as possible.

The reason why you are told not to eat bread, rice, pasta and other types of starchy carbohydrates is because your body is taking in and processing food differently after surgery.

The food absorption process changes after the Gastric Bypass procedure and your stomach is about the size of an egg. It is for after other weight loss procedures as well. Pasta, rice, bread are all very filling and take time to breakdown and digest. If you can imagine filling an egg with pasta or another carbohydrate I've mentioned, it's not much and will certainly not give you all the nutrients you need to survive. *Sticking to proteins* is a much better alternative in the months following weight loss surgery.

You will eventually be able to eat small amounts of most foods and you will quickly find out which ones will give you immediate discomfort and others that take so long to digest that they are not work eating.

I have realized that there are foods I've eaten that feel this way and Heaven knows I can't drink liquids to wash them down, so, I have to let my body process them naturally and it takes time.

The strange thing about certain foods after weight loss surgery is that sometimes you can eat them and other times you cannot. For me, I call this a *good food day* versus a *bad food day*.

Often if I am in a colder climate, stressed, nervous or in a hurry, it's never a good day to try to eat certain foods that my body tends to reject or that take a long time to process. Likewise, I know that when I am relaxed, sedate and usually in my quiet zone, I am remarkably able to eat lots of different things.

We already have discussed emotional eating as a food addict. I have to keep it in check at the relaxed times as I've noticed this is when I tend to overeat. As a food addict, because you have surgery doesn't change the fact you have a compulsion for food. *This will never change.*

It is how you monitor yourself that will keep you from harm's way. *Know your triggers and make sure that you are being honest with yourself.* Plan accordingly.

The one good thing for me and, hopefully it will be for you, too, is that stressful situations like parties or events won't allow you to overeat anymore because your body won't allow it.

Late at night, though, where we've all been hundreds of times before, watching TV, reading or just relaxing to music is when the nibbling begins.

Emotional grazing or nibbling can be dangerous and you need to have a *healthy nibbling alternative plan.* This is a perfect time to have a protein shake if you are in your beginning phase (or any phase), nuts or take a walk.

For me, I tend to have issues eating in the daytime with my schedule and have had to drink a Protein shake to fill me up so I don't crave food later at night. My body is used to certain foods now, six years after surgery and I've settled on a more *soft food diet* in lieu of meat and heavier foods.

I do like my snacks but instead of the more fatty chips I often have popcorn or sometimes salad croutons to get that *crunch* that we all seem to crave.

It was almost four years post-surgery when I started eating either of these foods. Every body is different. What works for some, won't for another.

You will need to sort out your personal routine that allows you to stay balanced to be successful. In the beginning and for at least the first 2-3 years afterward, you must follow the weight loss program and gradually start to introduce other types of food.

It is going to be challenging as you won't have eaten these foods in a while and your body won't be used to digesting them as easily, but don't get discouraged! Keep trying! Sometimes people ask me if I miss eating certain foods. Usually I tell them that sometimes the thought crosses my mind but, it's been so long that I don't even think about it anymore.

I actually haven't had a burger meal in over since the first week in March, 2008, over six years ago. My last burger was at Johnny Rockets which is strange since I probably ate fast food three or four times a week for over twenty years! *I've eaten it all before* and that's what you should be thinking if you get a craving or desire to stray off course.

You have eaten it all before! What did it get you? It got you to the point that you are now considering or have had a medical procedure to alter your body. It got you sick and unhealthy and has kept you from the quality of life that you deserve.

Stop and think about it. You are strong and you can do this. You have the ability and the courage to succeed.

If you don't think you can, then, there are groups
for support, therapy, your minister, friends,
family and of course you can contact
www.abundantlifearchitects.com for any special
help you need.

There's a great many who support you and are
rooting for your success as you say *no* to the foods
that have been holding you back in life and
keeping you off balance.

Tip #10: Mental & Physical Issues

When I decided to have weight loss surgery, it was after many painful years of yo-yo dieting, exercising, going to programs to lose weight and reading practically every self-help book on keeping weight off and living a happy lifestyle.

I had many people begging me not to have surgery, telling me I could die and saying if I just committed to a weight loss program and stuck with it that I would no longer be overweight.

Could *you* tell a drug addict or alcoholic they didn't really need inpatient treatment for their addiction but if their just *cut back* on their consumption and went to a 12-Step meeting once in a while they could live a drug free life? Of course you could not!

Now, let's change the scenario. You have a family member that needs medicinal marijuana for lower back pain they sustained while in the military on active duty in Iraq. They are addicted but need this to avoid the pain. Or, how about someone else that needs narcotic prescription pain medication and has also become addicted? They need their prescription.

These persons are *emotionally dependent on these drugs to cure their physical pain* in the same way you, the food addict, compulsively use substances (food) *like a drug* to cure your emotional problems.

A food addict is in pain the same way as the other examples and telling them just to diet and exercise as the solution isn't solving the problem. As you see, there are deep-seated psychological roots that cause any addiction and food is no different.

If you are struggling with any type of addiction before or after weight loss surgery, I urge you to seek out professionals who can help you to get these resolved as you need to address these issues before undergoing any surgical procedure.

It is imperative that you be honest with yourself about your reasons for having weight loss surgery. Surgery is not a magic wand that will take away your pain.

In fact, you might feel even worse after surgery. Perhaps the walls you have built for yourself by being overweight might no longer physically be there but the *emotion* behind the walls will remain until you make a choice to resolve these internal emotional barriers.

You will start out on Cloud 9 after weight loss surgery. Everything will be wonderful as the pounds start to melt off over the first six months if you are working your program as advised by your medical professional and weight loss center.

These are great reasons to celebrate while you get into different wardrobes, clothes and sizes you might have only dreamt of as a fantasy.

Doing the most ordinary little things in the world like walking up a flight of stairs instead of taking the elevator or even fitting comfortably in your car will soon amaze you. Maybe you can travel on a plane for the first time without buying a second seat, using an extender seat belt or fitting in the tiny restroom. Perhaps you can sit at a booth in a restaurant instead of sitting on a chair.

For me, it was not having to go to Big and Tall to purchase clothing and going to a brand name store for the first time in 3 years. This was a huge milestone! Please celebrate these monumental achievements because you deserve them!

You must also be knowledgeable that your body is physically shifting. There are chemical and physiological changes occurring as your body starts to adapt to the new you.

Since I'm not a doctor, I can't speak to why this happens, I just know it happens. Please consult your professionals that can help you best understand what is happening.

As a mentor and personal coach, I will tell you that your mind and different emotions are going to

take you on some pretty wild roller coaster rides
for a few years!

This is why is is extremely important that you
take your protein shakes, vitamins and
supplements, exercise and tell your doctor
everything that is happening.

Most weight loss surgeons and clinics don't ask lots
of questions about your mental status so make
sure you let them know so they can refer you if
you are needing someone to talk to about your
life.

This is a big life adjustment. People having this
procedure are losing sometimes a fully-grown
adult's body weight. Earlier, I wrote about the
mind and body needing to catch up and really
recalibrate itself to the new weight levels so this is

a time to make sure you are also resting as much as possible.

I had a CPAP for breathing due to Sleep Apnea and terrible snoring when I was heavy but after about 2 years I didn't need this any longer so I had to be sure I got very restful sleep.

It's all about balancing and creating the harmony that will keep you peaceful as your body goes through these radical changes.

You must also be patient with plateaus and your weight which will stall at various times, sometimes for weeks. This is your body getting accustomed to a new weight and it is recalibrating (balancing). If not, then, you are not following your weight loss plan. It's that simple.

I had at least two or three periods over two years where I went a few weeks without losing but I was prepared and knew to keep going with my plan. The same goes for you.

Don't get discouraged by plateaus and think of these as the body *resting* before getting going again. Stick to your routine and things will start moving again soon!

Over the years, I've had hundreds of people compliment me on my success and at first this praise felt so incredible. Over time, I started to get depressed and I couldn't understand why I felt that way when people said, *you must be so happy*. I felt like I was again lying like I did when I was in the grips of my food addiction and this was very dangerous.

During this process I also bought a house, ended a 6 1/2 year relationship with someone who did not support my weight loss goals, changed positions in my company and started working from home instead of in an office. Basically, I had multiple life issues to contend with alongside my weight loss program.

I also began to seek out risky people and more dangerous situations than ever before. This led to some reckless behavior at times as I was trying to find other addictive behaviors to fulfill what I no longer could satisfy with food.

You will need to look deep inside to see if you have any psychological or physical issues that might cause you to struggle after weight loss surgery because your mind will be wanting to feed its addiction in any way it can along your journey.

I was lucky in many respects but very unlucky in other aspects of my food addiction.

Thankfully, over six years post-surgery, I am in a comfortable spot and I am able to help others along their path. It's not only about losing the weight. It is preparing for a new life that will start to reveal itself the moment the emotional and physical healing begins.

You have done your research and you most likely have spoken with friends, watched, read or heard horror stories about the *physical issues* associated with weight loss surgery. Depending on the surgery, yes, you will have physical issues from time-to-time and since I am not a medical professional, I cannot speak to all of the types nor would I know as everyone is different.

I can tell you that if you don't follow your program precisely as you are told, you will get sick. The severity of physical illness depends on several things. I am advocating for a well-balanced lifestyle to be successful along your new life path.

For your *physical well-being*: protein shakes, water, vitamins and supplements, foods that are allowed on your new plan, exercise, rest, staying mentally healthy and *talking to your medical professionals* about what's going on with you are the keys to success. If you follow these steps, you should be able to avoid most physical problems.

For some, temporary hair loss will occur, you can get a hernia, headaches, various body ailments, stomach upset, throwing up, exhaustion, dehydration and vitamin deficiencies. You can also have many more serious complications, new addictions can develop and depression can occur.

Virtually all of these can be resolved by speaking honestly with your medical professionals and weight loss program immediately at the the first sign of any physical problems or symptoms. I cannot emphasize more that I have that talking to your doctor is vital to your success after weight loss surgery.

My Vitamin D deficiency actually led to a depressive episode and I needed to take medication for a couple of years. I was also dehydrated in another period of my weight loss and needed to increase my fluid intake.

At times, it seemed like nothing would stay down without me getting sick and I realized that my Lap

Band was too tight. I had to have it loosened (an adjustment fill removal) three times to be more comfortable.

While I didn't love going to the doctor every month for over 3 years, I did appreciate the results and it kept me honest, balanced, focused and committed. I hope the same happens for you and that you can embrace these great life events as the months and years pass!

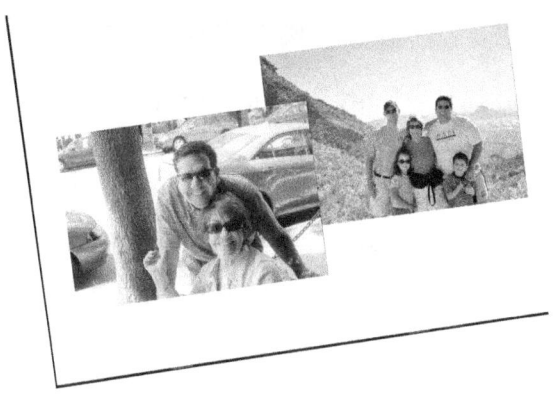

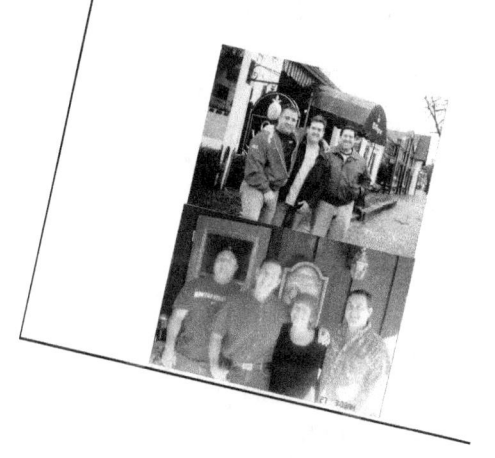

My family was very important

in my goal attainment.

Photos from Before and After.

Tip #11: New Ways to Cope

Learning new ways to cope after weight loss surgery is important. While *your* life has dramatically changed, the world around you, except for those who live with you, won't have shifted very much.

It will be very stressful at times for you as you experience the real world again living as a food addict after weight loss surgery. Good things as well as bad things can be equally hard to deal with for simple things like going to an event, dinner or cocktail party, eating out at a restaurant or traveling.

I wish I had a magic wand to shield you from any angst or grief but unfortunately I do not have this wand, so you'll need to be strong and find ways to handle these new types of situations as you get to learn how your new body functions and adapts.

I will focus on a few situations that are stressful but by no means is this a full list. I suggest you speak with local support groups for ideas. You can also email my website for any help along the way if you are seeking some mentoring or coaching sessions.

The first thing you need to learn as a person with a food addiction is the word *no*. Most of us are good, polite people. We were taught that money doesn't grow on trees and we needed to eat everything on our plates.

Some of us couldn't leave the table until we finished everything. People that are overweight don't want to hurt people's feelings and we also don't want folks to know we are secretly eating our emotions. We become great at pretending at the family picnics and all other functions by saying we are full.

Let's start thinking in reality now, OK? You are 75, 100, 150+ pounds overweight. *Do you honestly think people really believe you are not hungry?* Even if you aren't?

This is my Big Mac, with Large Fries and the Diet Coke Theory. I used to tell myself I didn't like the sugar because the sugar would make me fat but always wondered at the Drive Through Window what the staff thought when handing me my Big Mac Super-Sized meal with a *diet* soda.

I mean, who's kidding who? In fact, I used to eat a salad for lunch with coworkers, a nice healthy portion and then stop off at McDonald's for two Double Cheeseburgers to nibble on my way home from work before getting home for dinner! This is active food addiction.

I used to rationalize my behavior by saying I was under lots of stress at work but was only hurting myself.

Learning to say *no* is a must if you are going to deal with the stresses that will be coming along with your *weight loss surgery meal deal*. I promise you this one doesn't come super-sized, with fries or with a diet soda!

Saying *no* doesn't have to be mean or derogatory. People will understand your limitations as they see you progress over the months. It will be hard in the beginning as it is nearly impossible to eat the most foods, even tiny portions in most cases, because you either cannot, should not or won't as they will cause you to get off track.

Honesty is always best and it will free you from the stresses of having to attempt to do something you know is not in your best interest.

Eating at a Restaurant was probably the most tricky for me initially. I love dining out and love being with other friends, family and coworkers enjoying a nice experience. After surgery, this changed. I did go out to eat after a few months but learned eating anything new or different could not happen because I would usually get sick.

Eventually, I found spots that had nice soups since soup worked well for me and it was safe. You need to be prepared to take lots of items home if you dine out. I rarely get meals anymore and usually stick to soup or an appetizer. Bringing things home becomes costly and wasteful.

In the beginning, you will soon learn that the portions most restaurants provide are beyond anything you can tolerate in one meal post-surgery. It is really not worth it, even though your mind will be telling you to try to have the food. Just say *no*.

An interesting thing I found at restaurants and with virtually all servers was that when I first had surgery and asked for a *To Go Box*, the server usually gave a sad face and said, *Oh, you don't like your meal?* Society has conditioned us, just like you know the person at the McDonald's drive through window thinks, that heavy people are always hungry and if they don't eat something is wrong.

Now, fast forward 3 years to the same restaurant with the same server but I am now 163 (and had lost 160 pounds). I looked pretty thin. I wasn't hungry as the Lap Band was doing the same as when I weighed 330 pounds. The server said the same thing!

You might think this to be a coincidence but what if I told you that, In between, when I was very average that very few servers questioned me if I liked my food, rather, they simply provided the take away box?

I think if you are at either end of the spectrum you are suspect.

I recommend that you let your server and other dining guests know upfront that you have some dietary restrictions and most likely will need to take your food home.

For the pushy server that *affectionately* tells you that the portion you are ordering is very small (because you are very big at the time), well, tell them you had weight loss surgery and have to eat small portions. That usually does the trick!

Traveling and especially **traveling for work** can be challenging if you do not adequately prepare. First, you must let anyone you travel with know of your limitations, restrictions and that if you cannot keep up or do what they are doing that it is perfectly fine.

As I progressed, I could do things I never dreamed like hiking Little Mt. Sai in Washington which was something I couldn't do before because of the weight restriction and the feeling when I could was incredible.

I do recommend you speak with your doctor before planning any major trips and limit your travel in the first six months because you really need to get used to a consistent routine.

Travel is disruptive to your weight loss program and takes a good amount of planning to make sure you stay on track. It also takes you out of your comfort zone and opens the door to the emotional eating patterns you are changing as you work to understand your food addiction.

When you do travel, it is important you take along your essentials like protein shakes, vitamins/supplements and other foods that you know you can eat. If not, you might be sick or lose energy. You should also familiarize yourself with the local medical facilities should you need these during your travels.

Work Functions and Business Meals can be tricky. I was in sales and it was expected to have lunches and business meals. Some clients I knew before surgery, others had no idea and others would not have known as I was at an average weight when I met them.

In every instance, I told folks upfront that I had weight loss surgery and that my food intake was restricted and I apologized in advance if I didn't eat much (or at all). Everyone understood and it usually led to a friendly discussion about my weight loss program.

I told them weight loss surgery had changed my life in wonderful ways and I was pleased with my decision. I did not get into all the details and nor should you.

Keep it simple, honest and then proceed ahead as you would at any other function. Be sure you have a protein shake *before* the meal. Then, if you cannot eat due to stress, the types of food, etc., you won't have a grumbling stomach at the table or have to use your *exit plan* like I mentioned in Tip # 8 to find a restroom!

First Dates or folks that don't know about your surgery can present some stressful situations. We, as people who have hidden the truth from others behind our food addiction, are not as versed in the art of being upfront with others and telling them the truth.

After weight loss surgery, I decided to no longer be ashamed. At my first meeting I would talk about the elephant in the room and tell folks I was a food addict. I suppose it isn't much different than an alcoholic telling someone they don't drink. You need to do what makes *you* feel comfortable in your own time.

For me, I usually wait for an appropriate time in the conversation and then say used to be very heavy and had weight loss surgery and ultimately I lost about 130 pounds.

That's all I say unless I am talking with others who have had or are considering having weight loss surgery. I don't volunteer much more information as this really is my past life experience and it is not my current life.

By owning my past, I could let it go gently and I encourage you to do the same as you progress in your own life plan.

As a remembrance of my past, and, with a little prodding, I have been known to show people the two pairs of pants I kept (with a 52 inch waist). Most folks gasp when they see just how large those pants were compared to my 34 inch waist today.

Now I am at an average weight for my age that is comfortable for *me*. I don't look like a super-model or a college student in their twenties but that's just fine. It has taken me years to get my mind, spirit and body back in sync with a normal rhythm and balance.

It will take time for you, too. I didn't think it would take as long as it did, so be patient. I am now able to cope and handle just about any type of stressful situation that comes my way and not return to food for comfort or emotional support. You will see that you will be like me as long as you stay the course on your weight loss and life plan. Don't give up!

The family can eat it but you cannot is another one that can be difficult. I was single for most of the time post-surgery so I had more control over my daily routine and what I ate except when I was on a vacation or business trip.

I limited myself on meals out with friends, often didn't go to certain events that would cause issues with food or emotional eating and, at holiday's, everyone knew that I could only eat a very small portion.

Many of you have families that won't follow your same weight loss program and that is hard. Regardless if you have surgery or are just on a supervised weight loss program, *it's important your family all start to eat differently* as part of your overall weight loss plan.

You should speak to a nutritionist, support group or medical professional for advice before you begin your weight loss program.

With that said, you already know very well that buying Pop Tarts or serving Domino's Pizza to the kids a few times a week while you drink Protein Shakes is not the healthy alternative you are seeking. Talk to others in support groups or at your weight loss program if you have a family. It's really important for the whole family to support one another to have a balanced existence that allows for flexibility.

Not-so-helpful **friends, family or coworkers that allow you to fail** does happen and if you think it won't happen you are mistaken. I was honest with everyone after weight loss surgery about my goals and if they didn't want to support my new way of life and eating habits, they wouldn't be in my life. I stuck to this plan.

My family was very supportive but lived 1,500 miles away. My co-workers all knew and cheered me on which was fantastic. The office actually started having *healthy* potlucks and snack foods which was great. Most of my friends were supportive as well.

Unfortunately, my partner of 6 1/2 years liked the larger version of me and went so far as to say they were no longer attracted to me now that I had lost weight! I now realize how awful and self-destructive that was to my morale.

Luckily, I had many other people rooting for my success. Nothing was going to stop me from moving forward and, likewise, *nothing should hold you back or stop you from your plans* after weight loss surgery.

There will always be folks that are jealous of your success and this is inevitable. As you start to look different, act different, dress different and as your general demeanor changes, there will be folks who attempt to make you feel bad or knock you down. *Don't let them.*

Keep reminding yourself that this is all about you, your new life and your new pattern of thinking.

It's no longer only about weight loss. It is also about setting yourself free from the burdens and stresses of your food addiction. Think of your old emotional eating patterns melting away along with the pounds.

This is also helpful when someone says you should try some type of food or drink which you know is not on the approved list. Friends may tempt you but you do not have to agree and give in as this is an old pattern of behavior. Remember that powerful word *no*. It must become a strong interjection as needed and can be used politely to express your new found strength and balanced lifestyle.

Always carry healthy snacks and liquids as these will keep you out of harm's way in situations you cannot control. I toted around a small, insulated, plastic lunch sack with me for more than two years after surgery.

In this, I kept several of my 4 oz containers filled with different types of mini-meals and I tried to eat 1 or 2 oz portions at various intervals throughout the day. I also carried my 20 oz shakers that were pre-measured with my protein powder so I could just add water and shake!

Personally, I like cottage cheese, cheese cubes, pickles, shaved lean meats, soups and other soft foods so I kept these handy after I had my protein shakes if I got hungry. More often than not, I took these home as I simply could not eat much in the first six months.

Eventually I modified my meal planning as you will, too. To be safe, though, I made sure I had healthy snacks to munch on when I felt hungry. I also kept these in my car if I was at an event and couldn't eat the food.

It may be hard for you to believe right now but in my life right now I actually have to make sure I set aside time to prepare food and eat. Once you have surgery and start to heal your food addiction, as the years go by, food will take on a different meaning. *Eating food will no longer be emotional.*

Instead, you are will be eating to keep your body functioning properly and balanced.

Whereas before, eating was my sole purpose to attain emotional satisfaction for the pain I felt inside. *I lived to eat.* After years of self discovery and understanding the reasons behind my food addiction, I now *eat to live.* To accomplish this, I must set a routine that keeps me eating about six small meals each day.

I am reminded of many times that I planned everything I did around the next meal. On vacations, everything revolved around where we went to eat and we planned meals before anything else. I never thought a day would come that I wasn't thinking about food and then didn't eat!

It does happen and eventually it will happen to you a few years after weight loss surgery, so be aware that you have to plan to eat. This is my own plan and what works for me in *my* daily routine. You will develop your own plan as your body, and life, changes. Enlist the support of others, including your healthcare professionals, to help.

Keep in mind, eating food won't make you regain your weight. Your addiction to foods that are no longer good for you and which trigger an emotional reaction, *will*.

If you do not keep your food addiction under control, eating these types of foods again after weight loss surgery can send you on a downward spiral if not resolved immediately.

Programs like Overeaters Anonymous and Food Addicts Anonymous can help you. I often pop into a meeting to gain perspective, share and hear other stories that help me as a recovering food addict. You can also seek out professional counseling which is quite beneficial.

You may also find it useful to speak with a mentor or life coach like myself that specializes in working with people who have had weight loss surgery.

My greatest gift is being able to help others who are struggling with their weight and sharing my story. You *can* do this and if you've come this far, stay on the journey.

Life in balance after weight loss surgery is worth it . *You* are worth it!

Tip #12: Shapeshifting

After approximately 50 pounds of weight loss, you will need to buy new clothes. It varies from person to person, however, you should plan that as your body shape changes, so will your wardrobe.

I shopped at bargain basements and really liked The Goodwill Store which I shop at even today. These types of stores offer fantastic, name-brand bargains on gently used clothes. When you need to buy all new clothes every three months for about the first two years after weight loss surgery, you will want to look for special deals and the *colored tag days* will seem like a new best friend.

Yes, I have bought clothes off the rack at name brand stores but I actually find it more fun to look for hidden treasures at discount locations. You will decide what works for you and the best fit for your budget.

What goes along with your weight loss is also one of the most difficult things to mention: *excess skin* all over your body.

It is loose, wrinkled and very uncomfortable in the heat. After I had lost 100 pounds, I started to notice parts of my stomach that sagged almost as if it were hanging and I had to tuck it under my pants. I got very good at hiding the excess skin but it can exist on your arms, legs face, chest area and even your feet.

I had what I could only describe as a *waddle* under my chin that I hated. If you think getting your weight loss surgery approved is hard, try getting skin removal surgery paid for by insurance! It is something that has disturbed me for a long time.

People spend their lives obese and finally are committed to make a positive change, and when they do, the after-effects leave them feeling shamed again with a body that is disproportionate, saggy and unsightly.

I've told several people that the insurance companies should have folks who quality for weight loss surgery pay for a portion of the procedure depending on their ability to pay. Then, as an incentive to the insured for *literally* putting skin in the game, offer to pay for their skin removal surgery at 100% when they are medically cleared to have this procedure (usually after a person has lost over 45% of their original body weight and other conditions are met).

This is a life-changing surgery as people start to look like a real person again. This would be true wellness care. Considering how much an insurance company is paying annually for the overweight insured, this is a fraction of the lifetime costs of obesity.

I'm not here to get on my healthcare *soapbox*, so let's just say that you should be considering this second surgery if you desire and speaking with your medical professional after about one year after weight loss surgery.

It took me two years to be approved for skin removal surgery and I was denied the procedure the first time and had to literally *hold up my excess skin* in photos for the insurance company to show a rash that was under 10 pounds of excess skin around my stomach area.

I needed a Tummy Tuck and Abdominoplasty and happily made plans to have another surgical procedure. This surgery, though, was a much more difficult recovery.

I want to caution anyone going through skin removal procedures that this is an *extremely invasive surgery* and the surgeon is basically cutting your body apart to remove excess skin, tightening your abdominal wall and leaving you in staples and with drains for the fluid that builds up. My surgeon offered a tummy tuck and abdominoplasty at the same hospital and I trusted him so I decided this was the best course.

I knew I needed to take some time off work and went on company-paid disability for a month afterward. I mentioned stress in the previous tip and also discussed that life will change but you have to keep moving forward. I did what I could do to stay focused after skin removal surgery and keep a positive attitude during the months it took to fully recover.

In total, I spent two days in the hospital, had 10 *pounds* of skin removed, had 3 drains connected to my body for about six weeks after surgery, about 100 staples holding me together and a liquid Vicodin prescription for the pain. I was ready to tackle the world!

Recovery from skin removal surgery was difficult and much more challenging than the Lap Band surgical procedure. If you decide down-the-road to have skin removal surgery, you must prepare yourself for at least two months of recovery and honestly about four months to feel fully functional.

This is another major life decision and something you must talk through with your healthcare professional. Take it a step at a time and don't rush anything. In time, if excess skin removal surgery is what is best, it will happen.

Whether or not you have any type of surgery (weight loss or skin removal), after losing a considerable amount of weight your physical body will look very different. You will see yourself in the mirror and sometimes smile and might cry at other moments.

Think of yourself as beautiful no matter what shape you are shifting into along the road! I have never had my chin fixed or the excess skin removed from my chest area. Would I like to take care of this? Yes. Can I afford these procedures? No. I've made concessions and other adjustments along the way and used to say I would write a book someday to tell my story.

I am finally able to do this and to help others who are struggling. Life changes. *You* will change. It's all good and if you believe there is a purpose to your lifelong battle with weight and food addiction, then, you are way ahead of the game. I *know* you want to look and feel fantastic after losing so much weight. Try to be patient.

For now, perhaps, it's buying those designer jeans you never thought you could wear that will put a smile on your face. Maybe it's having some Botox injections. It could be a Tummy Tuck eventually, who knows. Whatever it is, it must be in balance

with your life goals and plan.

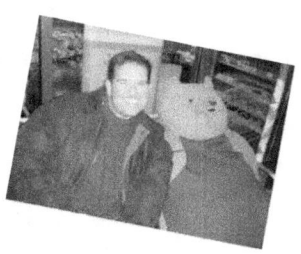

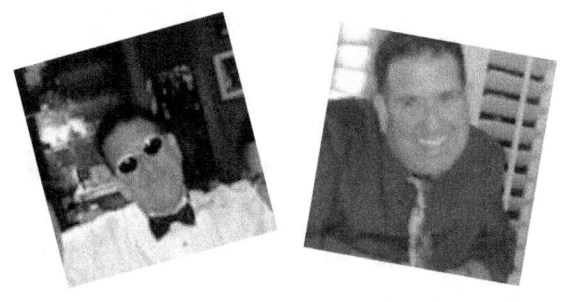

One, two and three years after

weight loss surgery.

Tip #13: Cheating

This is going to be a very simple discussion point: *if you are cheating on your program, you are only hurting yourself.* Before you decide to have weight loss surgery, you must ask yourself what you really want and what your expectations are after surgery.

I ask folks those questions when they approach me about having surgery and want to know what it is like. I tell them it is all about what you want to accomplish. Some people tell me they want to be healthy, more active and off their various medications. Others tell me they want to look wonderful.

Yet, some tell me they are *ready to change their lives forever and understand why food has controlled them.* These people, I am confident, are ready to embark on a new life plan because the surgery is only one part (weight loss). Overall, it is about *so much more* than simply losing weight. It's about *changing your emotional reactions to food forever* which will last a lifetime.

I've heard medical experts and some other professionals refer to weight loss surgery as a *tool* to help get you started. Most physicians also talk about proper diet and exercise to maintain the weight loss.

I'm not a medical professional but I *do* know many people who regain their weight after surgery. When this occurs, it's difficult to understand how someone committed to a new life would allow this to happen. It's food addiction and the emotional attachment to food that allows a person to compulsively overeat and regain their weight.

Sadly, a large number of people are either not prepared for the emotional challenges, don't have the support team needed, don't have the drive to succeed or simply don't want it enough. *Food addiction is a compulsive need to overeat due to emotional triggers and doesn't go away because you had weight loss surgery!*

If you have gotten this far in my story and have read the various tips I've given you, I hope you have been able to accept that food addiction has controlled your life. You must regain your power, not the weight and you must fight this emotional connection with food before it's too late.

A close friend of mine told me the story of his father-in-law that had the Gastric Bypass surgery and died only a few months later of heart failure. It was devastating to his family as he had wanted to do something about his being 250 pounds overweight for many years and then, when he finally did, he died.

I made the decision to pay for the procedure with my own money and a loan from my mother because I knew I couldn't wait any longer. I made the decision knowing my company was going to be bought out in a couple of months and we would have excellent health benefits that covered weight loss surgery. I made the decision *because I wanted to live.*

If you can fathom a remote thought of not wanting to live after weight loss surgery, then, cheat all you want. I am being blunt as *this is a matter of life and death*. This surgery is *not* cosmetic. Your body is a ticking time-bomb, riddled with future medical complications. Your quality of life will be non-existent if you don't start taking control of yourself *today, not tomorrow - today*.

I often remember watching the first year of the series The Biggest Loser. First, I hated the name as I thought it suggested heavy people were *losers*. I found myself drawn to this show, laughing, crying and identifying with contestants at every turn.

What was most ironic was during two of the seasons I was on a medically supervised weight loss plan trying to get approved for my first attempt at weight loss surgery in 2006.

I would sit and eat my salads while working out on one week and another week eating 3 double cheeseburgers (with no buns to follow the Atkins Carb Free Diet) with Vitamin Water (before I discovered their sugar content).

Was I cheating? Maybe not but I clearly was not ready to make a change in my life forever at that time. Sacrifice is never easy. I'm glad I made the changes and hope you are too!

Another memory of my personal cheating was working out at the gym and then going out with my friend to eat dinner at Friendly's Ice Cream! After spending an hour at the gym at 300 pounds, you bet I was hungry. What did I do? She and I would then go eat Bacon Cheeseburgers, Fries with a Diet Coke (of course) and then have a

Happy Endings Sundae. I wonder how many calories that negated from my workout? She also was very heavy and ultimately had a successful Gastric Bypass surgical procedure several years after mine.

I remember little kids staring and pointing at us and I felt so ashamed of how I looked. This is the horror and shame that we all have lived with for years as food addicts. I went to do something good by going to the gym and what did I want afterward? Yep, you got it. I wanted to celebrate with immediate gratification through food.

Are you beginning to understand the bigger picture of how food is part of *your* life?

The bottomline is we are all human and I am sharing some of my most personal stories to let you know I have been where you are far more than I'd like to admit.

If you are going to be successful in any type of weight loss program, you are going to have to *start by being honest with yourself*. Only then will you see that cheating is really another way for you to punish and shame yourself through your addiction.

Your brain tricks you, though. It tells you as a food addict that if you do something good you need to reward yourself with food like I did by celebrating with ice-cream. *This* is why people regain their weight. A food addict will think and rationalize things in their mind like *Ooooh, now*

I've lost 100 pounds, let's go to TGI Friday's and celebrate!".

You know you've done it. We all have done these self-destructive things to ourselves. So just stop the madness and start celebrating your new live in more balanced, healthy ways.

Susan Powter's excellent book Stop the Insanity from the early 1990's inspired me when I was only about 45 pounds overweight with her story. I am writing this for a reason to point out that I hadn't a clue about food addiction or the reasons why I would overeat.

Her book was no-nonsense approach to eating and living. I remember her writing something like *eat when you are hungry and drink when you are thirsty*, which absolutely makes sense and is something I will discuss in Tip # 15.

Unfortunately, I wasn't ready to deal with my food addiction, so all the self-help books did me no good and ultimately led me to the surgeon thirteen years later.

Similarly, in Oprah's book Make the Connection, I cried and howled at her descriptions of all the diets she tried and her yo-yo process over years of trying to lose weight and keep it off. I was on the Atkin's diet a few years later and remember her writing to *remember the breath mints* because the protein only diet makes your breath smell nasty. Also, that *sometimes you just want a piece of bread*! Here I am today to tell you that Oprah was incredibly accurate.

Ordinary diets and exercise won't work, long-term, for a food addict without understanding the emotional aspects behind eating. When you are prepared to accept this as fact, you will be ready to make a change in your life forever.

If you or another person you know suffers with any type of addiction, this will sound familiar. *Until you are ready to admit you are powerless over food, food will continue to control you.* Make no mistake, long after surgery food will still have the power to control everything you if you allow this to happen.

You do not have to continue in this pattern. At a point in your weight loss program and after surgery, the light will come on and you will realize this is not only about weight loss, *it is about your ability to take control over your life again* and not allow yourself to be a victim of food addiction anymore. It's about you being able to confidently look at yourself in the mirror and say, *I am worth it!* Because, you *are* worth it!

Let's make a pact together right now, OK? *No cheating.* Cheating on your weight loss plan can mean many things to different people but, for the sake of simplicity, we will define cheating as *not following your weight loss program as directed by your medical professionals.* Your plan should be monitored by a medical professional and their team.

You will be provided with a very specific list of foods that you are not allowed to eat after weight loss surgery. Can you agree that you won't eat them? Eating foods that are not recommended in your new lifestyle would be a deliberate attempt to harm yourself and would be an old pattern in your food addiction.

Your *no no* list is given to you by your weight loss reason and it is not to make you suffer, it is to assure that you live a happy life after weight loss surgery. Eating these foods will stall your weight loss, make you sick and, in the worst scenario, cause you to regain weight.

Foods that are high in refined sugar content tend to *slide down* and digest much easier. For the Lap Band patient, eating or drinking high calorie foods like ice cream or milkshakes (that pass through with little or no restriction) is called *cheating the band*. Just say no like I talked about in Tip #11.

The last thing I want to mention about cheating is that people can't get inside your mind and body. If you don't tell the truth about what is going on, you are cheating.

If you describe to your physician, for example, the Lap Band is too tight when you *know* you want it looser so you can eat more food, this is also cheating. Not disclosing foods you have eaten that are either restricted or frowned upon is cheating.

Think of this as one of your biggest challenges and be honest with yourself first. Then, be honest with everyone else around you. If you are like I was, I am certain that most of you haven't been truthful with yourself or anyone else for many years. These lies you tell yourself and others have led to your current life's circumstances.

If you don't cheat, you will stay balanced. If you stay balanced, you *will* achieve success. When you are successful, you will start to enjoy a very satisfying lifestyle post-surgery. You will also no longer be cheating yourself out of a happy life and paralyzed by food addiction.

Tip #14: Substituting Addictions

If you are considering weight loss surgery or any type of serious program to lose weight, most medical professionals will tell you that you should cut out alcohol and to be very aware of prescription and non-prescription drugs.

First and foremost, remember that you are a food addict, *you have an addiction* and it is very easy to migrate to a multitude of other addictive behaviors as your body starts to change and your brain chemistry shifts.

You are making a commitment to change your life forever and in doing so you will need to take a careful inventory of other demons that may be lurking in that closet filled with all the pain and suffering you have likely endured most of your life until now.

There are many articles out there about people who become drug addicts or develop alcoholism after weight loss surgery. There are other stories of people developing other types of addictions as well.

From what I've read, food addiction seems to be the most prevalent in the pleasure center of the brain. When someone who is used to getting pleasure by eating food (their addiction) and is then deprived of this through weight loss surgery, the food addict's brain will often seek other means to satisfy themselves (their pleasure center) through drugs, alcohol and even sex.

Remember, the brain is working on high alert after weight loss surgery to process out all the fat, toxins and re-calibrating toward a balanced body chemistry. As you have always used your pleasure center of the brain to satisfy your food addiction, they brain chemistry is now altered by denying food for pleasure.

Often, without even knowing it, your brain works overtime trying to find a way to re-balance itself and waits for the opportunity (or creates an opportunity) to achieve that balance through other means.

Re-calibrating your body will take several years after weight loss surgery. In the meantime, if left unchecked, the mind can wreak havoc on a person as I have mentioned here and also Tip # 10 regarding emotional and physiological changes.

This information may be overwhelming to you and I am only touching on the subject but you must be aware at all times of your susceptibility to substitute one addiction for another. You should seek out professional help immediately if you feel in any way that you are substituting addictions. This is a time to be honest with yourself!

I've always been outspoken, boisterous and like to have a good time when I am at play. I was, of course, told by my weight loss program to be very careful about drinking alcohol after weight loss surgery as I wasn't eating as much food and my tolerance level would be much lower.

At first, it seemed fine to have a few drinks on the weekend after surgery but I was still quite large at the time. As I started losing more weight, friends would tell me I was louder and my personality was different when I drank. I didn't understand this as, to me, I seemed normal but wasn't. I would not eat before going out which was bad and I would then have 3-4 drinks in an evening. A few times I could not remember all the events of the evening which frighted me.

I started doing some investigating and realized one drink a person that had not had weight loss surgery could have the effect of three in mine! Please be very aware of everything you are putting in your body that is toxic (and, like alcohol, has lots of empty calories). Talk to your doctor, support group, counselor or others in different types of recovery programs to gain their perspective.

Some weight loss procedures don't allow alcohol after surgery as the body cannot tolerate it and you will be ill. *The brain doesn't know you you had weight loss surgery.* All it wants is to get back into balance that was disrupted when you deprived it's pleasure center of food.

Drinking alcohol, even though a depressant, tricks the brain at first by stimulating the pleasure center. Suddenly, it is satisfying it's craving for the pleasure it got before through food now with alcohol.

Whatever you decide to do is your choice, but I highly recommend curtailing or eliminating alcohol from your diet at least for a significant length of time post-surgery.

If you are on prescription medication, your weight loss surgeon needs to know how these are reacting in your body over time. Your specialists also need to be aware that you had surgery and your team of professionals may need to collaborate to make sure you are balanced in every aspect.

If you are taking non-prescribed drugs, like smoking marijuana or using other types of street drugs, please stop. If you feel you cannot control your behaviors and need help there is support 24 hours a day.

Call the 24 Hour National Helpline at 1-800-662-HELP (4357). This number supports all types of Substance Abuse and Mental Health related issues. It is confidential and free of charge.

The last topic I want to mention in this tip is sex. Sex is often difficult to talk about openly with people. Those of us with body image issues have hidden our bodies, kept the lights off and felt ashamed at how we looked. After losing weight, we are now suddenly thrust into the forefront to deal with emotions and attractions that many of us haven't considered an option for years.

For those already in relationships, you might have healthy sexual relations with your partner or your may not. Many persons have simply closed themselves off to love for fear of being hurt.

Others might have stopped having sex altogether. Still, there are other folks that use their large body images to attract people with fetishes for larger men and women for sexual gratification.

Regardless of where you fit in the spectrum, your attitudes, beliefs and values are going to change after you have lost a significant amount of weight. Even if you are single like I am today, I celebrate the many joys in my life and I am open to the possibility of a new, loving and committed relationship with someone that I can freely give love back to without fear or conditions. I haven't always been able to say this in the past.

With that said, your brain, in its search to satisfy the pleasure center, unfortunately may lead you to places that you never planned to go or into dangerous situations that you may regret.

I urge you to be aware of your thoughts and actions after weight loss surgery, especially after losing a significant amount of weight in a short period of time.

Being aware of your behavior, writing about it in your journal and talking to other professionals if you have concerns is quite important.

If you feel in any way you are engaging in unsafe practices or risky behaviors, take immediate action. As I mentioned before, you can call the National Helpline for guidance.

You can talk about this in support groups and with your medical or mental health professional. Spiritual guidance is often available. 12-Step Recovery Programs as well as friends and family maybe can helpful in sorting out any other addictive behaviors.

Exercise is a great way to release endorphins and to naturally stimulate the brain's pleasure center. Hopefully you can use exercise as a tool in your toolbox for years to come after weight loss surgery since this *also* tricks the brain as easily (and in a much healthier way) as alcohol, drugs or sex.

When you are able to better understand food addiction and how your body chemically reacts to food in your brain, it will be much easier for you to comprehend how easy it is for the brain to substitute addictive behaviors through alcohol, drugs and sex.

Thinking about this now is perhaps the first time you are putting a whole person together that is fully open, honest and functional. When you achieve this, you will feel amazing!

It's taken several years to get where I am now and who knows what is next but what I *do* know is

I am content. I made a commitment after weight loss surgery to take a very hard look at my life, my patterns and my addictions.

I hope you can be brave and strong to do the same thing now, deal with the addictive aspects and live a wonderful, balanced life!

Tip #15: Listening to your Body

As I mentioned in Tip #13 from Susan Powter's book Stop the Insanity, she mentions to eat when you are hungry and drink when you are thirsty which I wholeheartedly agree.

The only caveat which we talked about in Tip #7 about food intake is that your body might not be able to tolerate what you want, so you have to be aware of your portion sizes.

Yes, you may be thirsty but gone are the days you can chug down 24 ounces of liquid without stopping. Likewise, bolting your food like you are in a race or eating more than a couple ounces at a time is a sure recipe for major discomfort.

Your body will crave different things at different times. It will be somewhat odd to you I am certain, if you are like me, when your body suddenly wants something salty or sweet *but your mind is no longer saying donut or potato chips* as it did in the height of the food addiction.

Before weight loss surgery I mostly enjoyed starchy carbs, sauces and crunchy chips. I didn't usually like sweets or crave sugary items. So, imagine pastas with cream sauce, butter, potatoes, rice, corn, every type of chip and dip plus of course the burgers, pizza and chinese food!

After surgery, I started to crave sweets in a way I never had before which obviously meant I was depriving my system of these starchy carbohydrates that break down like the energy source for sugar in the body and store themselves as fat cells in the body.

Basically, the protein shakes were working and my fat cells were shrinking as the fat was needed for energy in my body to function. After I lost a significant amount of weight and had little fat stored in reserve to use as energy, my body was asking for it's energy source that I could not longer eat due to my weight loss surgery. I have to be careful when I get a sugar craving and so should you.

Occasionally, I get cravings for sodium and other times for ice cold water. Usually I get plenty of sodium in my diet through protein and other foods I eat and drink but it has occurred when I've been having more plain drinking water. I actually really enjoy plain water now. It really quenches my thirst.

Once in awhile I get a craving for a regular, sugary soda that actually provides me with the water, sugar and sodium! This is a rare occasion when I have regular soda but it meets my needs when my body says it needs these elements.

You will need to be aware that your body won't be in this state for a couple of years until you have lost all the weight. I am not advocating a specific diet that contradicts your program. I am letting you know, though, that down the road you will have certain requests from your body and should determine what it needs so it stays balanced and is operating at maximum efficiency.

I still do like crunchy snacks. I think this goes along with the food addiction and my brain's compulsion to want carbohydrates that crunch and are tasty (this means salty). Since I don't eat bread and haven't for six years, occasionally I munch on flavored croutons or crackers.

Rather than deny my body something it is obviously missing, I have tiny portions that I feed it when these urges arise. I still use my handy 4 oz containers to keep myself in check with portion control.

After more than six years post-surgery, I no longer drink 3 Protein Shakes a day, take all the vitamins and supplements I did in the first few years or follow the strict plan I originally did but this is to be expected. I get most of my calories from eating solid food and I need to feed it correctly so I have energy.

Eventually your body will be eating solid food but you always can fall back to one or two protein shakes a day to get back on track if you notice you are regaining weight.

If you notice when I mentioned cravings as part of understanding what your body is asking you for, I didn't mention I had a craving for blueberry pie, Krispy Kreme donuts or a Mars Bar. I said my body was craving sugar which is how carbohydrates break down as energy.

I didn't write I needed Pringles, a Bagel or The Olive Garden for pasta and breadsticks. I said sodium which is needed to help the functions for many systems in your body.

To keep your body in a balanced state, it needs to regulate various processes that require multiple vitamins, minerals, proteins, fats, carbohydrates amongst others to enter, be processed and this is how the body functions.

Most of the nutrients we need from food on a daily basis are available in things we commonly eat like fruits, vegetables/legumes, whole grains, proteins and dairy products. Several years after weight loss surgery you will still need these same nutrients to maintain proper health so keep this in mind.

I am not a medical professional and these are my personal views after going through weight loss surgery and living my life for over six year afterward. I'm not an expert as much as I am someone who has learned to understand what his body needs to function and to stay balanced.

Please consult *your* medical professionals for help in understand what your body will need to function in a balanced state.

I also know how my body reacts to food and foods that trigger my food addiction. The more *you* start to get to know your body and how it functions, the better off you will after weight loss surgery or any weight loss program.

If you body is exhausted, sore or depleted of energy, then, maybe change up your workouts. Be sure you are taking all your vitamins and supplements. Make sure you are properly hydrated.

Your body will be processing fat 24/7. If you cannot get out of bed in the morning, if you cannot fall asleep at night, if your are agitated or nervous, these *can* be signs of vitamin deficiencies, dehydration, stress or depression.

I've mentioned in this information in other tips. *Listen to what your body is telling you* and seek whatever personal or professional advice you need to keep your body well-balanced after surgery.

The same goes for eating. Your weight loss program might differ on this one so check with them but I have found eating six *tiny* meals a day works best and keeps me remembering to eat. I follow the same for fluid intake. I drink six to eight beverages a day which are either flavored water, diet soda or regular filtered water.

Sometimes there are days I have a mad craving to eat and other days I cannot eat anything. Other times, it's hard to get liquids down.

Cold temperatures for me or the start of the day tend to be more difficult to get food and fluids to go down. At night,though, I can get most food to process the way it should.

I listen to what my body is telling me to avoid complications. It is very important *you* do the same.

After a while, when you have moved well-beyond surgery and your first few years of maintaining your weight, you may be tempted on occasions to overindulge. This will happen and if you have had weight loss surgery, you most likely will be sick unless you after too much food intake.

For those with procedures like the Gastric Bypass, your stomach is elastic and, even while it was reduced to about a third of it's original size, after a year or two it expands as you attempt to consume larger portions.

This is how many people regain their weight. The same goes for people who graze on food all day often regain their weight. If you haven't dealt with the emotional aspects of eating, it will be very easy for your mind to play tricks on you and start you eating the wrong foods.

Therefore, it's important to beware if your body is telling you it needs something. It may actually be your brain wanting to self-soothe in order to cope with stress or life circumstances. *Control your portions, follow these 15 Tips* and

remember, *these are old patterns of behavior.*
Unfortunately, your food addiction will plague you
if you don't deal with it now.

Today, after six years post-surgery, if I become
sad or depressed, my brain isn't telling me it
wants a protein shake or to go to the gym. I
wish it did. Instead it says, *I want to eat a
grilled cheese sandwich with bacon with tomato
soup* and lay on the couch watching romantic
comedies on Netflix! Go figure.

Since I cannot eat the grilled cheese, what I do is
make tomato soup. I then add a few croutons
which I top with some shredded cheese and some
bacon bits if I have them. Voila, I have instant
gratification but in a much healthier way.

I am also more aware of my emotions, so, before I dive into the soup, I ask myself what is really going on and why I am feeling like this in that moment. I make the necessary adjustments and, sometimes this actually does become a trip to the gym or a walk outside instead of the movie laying on the couch. Or I go and do volunteer work. Or I write a letter to a friend.

I try to do proactive social activities *to keep shifting my mind away from the food needing to be the resolution for the emotion.*

This is difficult and has taken years of practice and work with other professionals and work with a life coach. I don't expect you to become an expert at this overnight but want you to be aware of the emotional aspects of eating and how your body reacts to these.

There are countless numbers of people out there to help you if you are struggling and I am only one opinion on this topic. I am one, though, who has had to work through weight issues and food addiction for over 40 years. I am very knowledgeable of my own triggers and those of other folks I talk to about weight loss and food addiction.

If you need individual support, email me at www.abundantlifearchitects.com and I will be happy to help!

The end is just the beginning.

Well, there you have it. These are my 15 Tips to staying balanced after weight loss surgery which have now been passed along to you. I am hoping through my story, you can identify with someone that shares in your struggles and understands your pain.

I know there are many difficult decisions to make if you decide to have a particular weight loss surgical procedure. These tips will help to get you started and guide you to the right resources and medical professionals to be sure you are getting exactly what is best for *your* unique situation.

Your needs might be greater than what I can provide in these 15 Tips. If this is the case, I urge you to use the various professional resource links I have provided to make sure you get the proper help you need. *Food addiction is serious. Obesity is an epidemic in the United States.*

Life is precious and so is *your* life! I hope as you have read these 15 Tips, you have been able to gain more confidence in yourself through my adventures.

Whatever you decide to do, make sure you cherish the body you were given, honor the wonderful person you are and love who you are on your life journey.

If you are ready to heal your food addiction and to start a whole new life, there are many who have been there before, with outstretched arms, ready to welcome you as you say goodbye to your past and start living again.

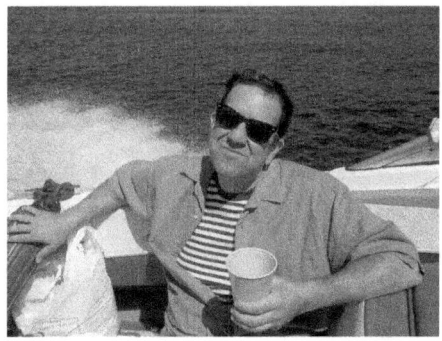

July 2011 - 173 lbs. - Living Again!